A must read for individuals and family members who are touched by cancer. It will be an eye opener for healthcare providers, such as nurses, doctors and allied professionals.
—Jame Abraham, M.D., FACP Bonnie Wells Wilson Distinguished Professor and Eminent Scholar; Chief, Section of Hematology-Oncology Medical Director, Mary Babb Randolph Cancer Center West Virginia University

Kevin wrote this book to help couples cope with the emotional side of this dreaded disease called cancer. But men—take heed. Read this book and learn that when cancer comes to you, your wife, or a family member, it is okay to pray, weep, and most important of all, seek help from others. This book will make a difference in your life.
—Dick Vitale, College Basketball Announcer

Get out your hankies, open your mind and heart to raw emotion — and profound life lessons. Kevin Murphy shares a very personal, intimate story of an evil disease that mercilessly stalks not just the body of a loved one—but invades and threatens everyone close by. Even the best relationships are tested, and some do not survive. He turns his own painful experience into deeply faith-based, inspirational lessons learned, in hopes that others are spared the suffering this hateful disease leaves in its wake.
—Judith G. Clabes, Editor and Publisher KyForward.com; Former President and CEO, Scripps Howard Foundation

I recommend this book not just to those suffering from cancer and their spouses, but also to my colleagues in the medical profession. As a physician who has interacted with cancer patients for close to 30 years, this book was an eye opener for me.

D1262544

How does one put into words the human experience of Cancer? Kevin Murphy has accomplished this by way of his personal journey and fight against the ultimate fear of losing a wife/ marriage, and ensuring the birth of two exceptional daughters. The emotional burden that Cancer places upon a marriage and family will certainly be minimized by reading this book and learning the evolution of change necessary to survive Cancer.
— Peter J. Ganshirt, Psy.D., Licensed Psychologist

This is a wonderful, heartfelt book to help cancer patients understand the strong emotions that come with this disease. As a chiropractor who has cared for many cancer patients over the years, I hope you read this story and stay connected to those you love.
—Dr. Cathy Gratkowski, Chiropractor, Florence Chiropractic Center

Surviving Cancer
After Surviving Cancer

Coping With the Emotional Side of Cancer

by Kevin L. Murphy

Foreword by Bernie S. Siegel M.D.

To Candace
Cancer can never
defeat love!
Kevin J Murphy

Headline Books, Inc.
Terra Alta, Wv

Surviving Cancer After Surviving Cancer
Coping With the Emotional Side of Cancer

by Kevin L. Murphy

To order additional copies of the book, or to contact the author:

Headline Books, Inc.
P O Box 52
Terra Alta, WV 26764

www.HeadlineBooks.com

For Further Information please visit:
www.KLMurphy.com

Cover concept by Kathleen Colón and Kevin Kelly

ISBN-13: 978-0-938467-40-3

Library of Congress Control Number: 2012936450

Murphy, Kevin
Surviving CancerAfter Surviving Cancer
    ISBN 978-0-938467-40-3

1. Cancer 2. Psychological 3. Relationships 4. Self-Help-- Non-Fiction

PRINTED IN THE UNITED STATES OF AMERICA

Foreword

"Loyalty is a precious quality that we have almost lost sight of today. Instead of loyalty, almost everyone talks about freedom, especially in relationships. The idea is that if two people come together in freedom, each can walk out of the arrangement. This is supposed to be a complete safeguard against unhappiness. But even where both are free to walk out – where there are no obligations, no bonds, not even any ties – they go on doing this over and over and do not acquire the capacity to love. Without loyalty, it simply is not possible to love deeply" (Eknath Easwaren).

When I first heard from Kevin Murphy via email about his book, I told him he was not a normal lawyer. I meant that as a compliment, because from my perspective, lawyers are trained to think and not to feel. But as you will see, Kevin is willing to share his painful experience and feelings, and the lessons he learned from them. Cancer has many side effects, and as you will learn from this book, not all of them are bad. They can become your teacher, and help you to heal your life and relationships.

Let me share a quote a lawyer sent me many years ago. He was involved in an emotional event while talking to a client in the street. Their conversation was interrupted because his client was told that his son was taken to the emergency room. He started to think about what to do with his client's car and the keys, and came to a *logical* conclusion about what to do with both. But then the light bulb went on. He realized what he really needed to do was to go to the emergency room. He said, "I came to a conclusion that was eminently reasonable, totally logical and completely wrong, because while learning to think I almost forgot how to feel."

Kevin is a lawyer who has the ability to feel, and wants to share those feelings and wisdom with everyone in order to help them avoid the pain he experienced.

Kevin would like to see the lessons he shares with you, especially the men, help you to live your authentic life, and reduce the need for divorce. However, divorce is not always a bad choice. As one woman I know said, after going through a mastectomy for breast cancer and a divorce, "I gave up a tit *and* an ass." When something threatens your health, it is best to eliminate it from your life. But otherwise, you should ask yourself how love can heal the relationship.

As a surgeon, I know how many find it so difficult to deal with the experience of pain and loss. But swallowing those feelings can and will become destructive. Joseph Campbell and my wife agree about marriage. Campbell described it as an ordeal, and my wife called it a struggle. Why? Because it is about a relationship, and not about the individual. In other words 1+1=3, which means two people create the third entity, the relationship, and relationships take work to create and maintain.

In my thirty years counseling people with life threatening illnesses, I have seen how hard it is for men to participate in support groups and share their feelings. Men are into doing and thinking and not feeling. I know men who, after a cancer diagnosis, considered or committed suicide because they couldn't work anymore, and felt there was no point in living. They would express these feelings while their wives and children were sitting right next to them, and hearing firsthand that they were not seen as reasons for living. It is a sad fact that most men refuse to support their wives when they are asked by them to attend their cancer support group. In my three decades of practicing medicine, I saw only six men show up and say that they were attending because they loved and supported their wives. A few others who attended would say only a curt comment like, "I'm her chauffeur." I actually met one loving husband who wrote a poem about being her chauffeur, realizing he was separated from his wife's reality by the glass partition, but yet still on the journey with her and ready to help her get to where she wanted to go.

Kevin writes that "cancer can devour the relationship." That is true, only if you let it. The problem isn't the cancer. The problem is the people involved in the marriage or relationship of any sort, whether it is the doctor and patient, teacher and student, or husband and wife. When we can listen to each other and coach each other through constructive criticism, then the relationship flourishes. As Helen Keller said, "Deafness is darker by far than blindness." When we listen to each other, we hear what is being said, and can know ourselves better. When you can accept criticism from those living the experience and not make excuses, you become a better spouse, doctor and teacher.

Many years ago, at the age of seven, one of our children told me his leg hurt and he needed an X-Ray. The X-Ray revealed a bone tumor, and the odds were that it was malignant, and that he had a year or so to live. I went home after seeing his film and tried to explain to my wife and our five children what was likely to happen to Keith. I thought it was appropriate that we all be depressed about the future. The next day Keith came to me and asked if he could talk to me for a minute. I said sure and he responded, "Dad, you're handling this poorly." This seven year old went on to tell me that they wanted to have a fun day, yet I wanted them all depressed in their bedrooms. He taught me a great deal in a few minutes. Fortunately, he had a very rare benign tumor, but I learned a lot before his surgery.

After having five children in seven years, including twins, my wife developed Multiple Sclerosis, and I spent a week in the hospital with a serious infection. We were exhausted and vulnerable, and learned we needed help. We started asking everyone from neighbors to my patients to help us, and they did. And as my wife later said, "They saved our lives."

Many years later she developed breast cancer, and I was impressed with what life had taught me, and how calmly I handled the cancer versus my previous problems confronting her MS and predictions about the future. I have learned from my experience and the wisdom of others that when love is involved there are no burdens. To quote my wife Bobbie, "I love you. You love me. Everything is alright." We have built our life with the bricks of love and held them together with the mortar of humor. We keep our inner child alive and participating in our lives, so we can enjoy the day and learn from each other. The future may be uncertain, but enjoying the day is our goal. Who knows what our potential may be!

It is by doing that we work at healing our lives and relationships and benefit from the results psychologically and physically. As Mother Theresa put it when asked to speak at an anti-war rally, "I will not attend an anti-war rally but if you ever have a peace rally call me." We need to choose life and work at healing our lives and relationships by finding peace, instead of fighting a war against cancer and divorce and empowering our enemy. Then our difficulties become our labor pains of self birth, and by giving birth to our new selves and new relationship, they become worthwhile.

The key is keeping our power and remembering the choices are ours and not the doctors. They can prescribe but we decide. Doctors are not trained in communication skills, so their wordswordswords become swordswordswords and can kill or cure like a scalpel. The phone calls to Kevin and his wife about having cancer show how poorly the medical profession understands the experience people are living versus their diagnosis.

When people do well they are told by their doctor to keep doing whatever they are doing. Instead the doctor should ask, "What are you doing that has kept you well?" There is survival behavior and Kevin tries to teach that in this book from his experience. They are simple things like having a sense of meaning in your life, asking for help when you need it, expressing appropriate anger, saying no to what you do not want to do, and using your pain as you would hunger to lead you to nourish your life and more.

When we learn from the wisdom and experience of others, we do not need to experience a disaster and write a book to enlighten others. Read what has been written and learn from the wisdom of the sages who have been where you now are. Then you don't ask God, "Why me?" Rather, you can confront God and say, "Try me!" It is also important to not let your beliefs make you feel God is punishing you or using a disease to make you more spiritual. When you lose your car keys, you do not assume God wants you to walk home. So when you lose your health, look for it as you would your car keys.

If you grew up with parents whose actions and words were destructive and gave you mottos to die by, you can abandon your past as part of the rebirthing of your self. Create new expression to live by, be assertive and let your heart make up your mind. You control one thing—your thoughts and feelings —which create your internal chemistry. So do not live a role but instead, an authentic life which will help you to find hope, love and faith to achieve your potential. Self-induced healing is a reality in your marriage and physical body. To have this happen you must quiet your mind and life to see your true reflection in the still pond. We are all swans. This is something Kevin struggled with throughout his experience with his wife's cancer—the inability to quiet his mind.

He did, however, act like a survivor in displaying action,

wisdom and devotion. He took steps to change things, was active in seeking information to help himself and his wife, and he had faith to sustain him. That is why I consider him to not be a normal lawyer.

Men have problems with relationships and need to do things rather than feel. Women live longer than men with the same cancers, as do married men compared to single men. It is because relationships give our lives meaning, from our pets to our families. The problem for men is asking for what they need. They need to learn that you are a success when you find peace, and it is okay to ask for someone to rock you to sleep and to stop doing things all by yourself, as a country western song tells us.

So if one door is slammed shut, you keep looking further down the corridor for the open door and let go of the guilt, blame and shame related to the illness and marriage. We are all wounded, and when we share our wounds, healing happens. It is harder for a lawyer to do this, but when you open your heart magic happens, because those who are wounded respond to you and your needs. As Thornton Wilder wrote, "In love's service only the wounded soldier can serve."

Angels appear, and there are no coincidences. My life and people's stories I share in my book *A Book of Miracles* reveal my beliefs and experience. They are attracted by our consciousness, and Kevin shares his experience here too. Their second child was a miracle. When we live in the moment and realize yesterday is dead and gone, and tomorrow is out of sight, then we help each other to make it through the night—and the darkness of our difficulties and miracles become a part of our lives.

So love your self, your body and your life, and miracles of healing will occur. This does not mean living in denial, but rather accepting your difficulties and asking for help. How God responds to your prayers depends on several factors. As the song says, "When you can't lean on no one else that's when you find yourself." So if you are in premature labor, God and others will step in to help you stop the labor. But when you are full term God steps back, because it is then time for you to step up and make the necessary changes for self-birthing. That is what Kevin is sharing in his book and lessons.

Creating your authentic self is not about becoming a human *doing* but becoming a human *being*. I hear women say to their kids, "I can't die until you're all married and out of the house." When the last kid leaves home Momma dies. Men die or commit suicide when they can't work anymore. It is about contributing love, not about what you can do and living a role. When you are authentic your life has meaning, and you are contributing love to the world in your chosen and unique way. Life is like a marathon and our job is to finish the journey we are on. Fear and failure are not the issue—they are self-destructive. It is all about taking responsibility and participating in your life that counts. So reach out and touch one another because a touch heals. Keep the child in you alive so that your relationship leads to a sharing of love and laughter. And remember, the only thing of permanence and which is immortal is love.

One last test which can help you in your relationship— how do other people seem to you? If you like people and see nice qualities in them it is because you have these qualities in you. If all you see are negative and troublesome qualities in others, you are projecting your problems onto them. If you want to maintain a relationship, accept responsibility for your behavior and personality and work at becoming the person you want to be. We are all actors, and your lifetime gives you the opportunity to rehearse and practice becoming the person you want to be.

To summarize my thoughts before you learn from Kevin's experience and wisdom, accept that life is difficult and relationships can be an ordeal or struggle, especially with cancer or other serious illness. Be willing to participate in the healing of each others wounds. Find coaches, learn from others and let their criticism polish your mirror and apologize when you hurt others.

Our darkest moments can become the charcoal which under pressure becomes a diamond, and like hunger, can lead us to nourish our life and relationships. Then the curse becomes a blessing.

Do not judge or advise unless you have lived the experience others are going through. Tourists do not understand what natives are living. So live the experience and do not intellectualize everything. Let the emptiness you feel become your womb and not your tomb. Let your labor pains give you a new life and become worthwhile.

In closing, learn from Kevin's book to kill with kindness, torment with tenderness, love yourself, your body and everyone in your life. Don't fight the enemy of divorce or cancer, but work at healing your life and relationships and serving love, so that everyone benefits no matter what the future holds.

Bernie S. Siegel, M.D.

INTRODUCTION

If you have picked up this book, odds are that you, a spouse or a loved one has or recently had cancer. I feel for you. There is no sugar coating it. It stinks. But you have no choice but to deal with it in the best way possible.

If just diagnosed, your doctors and technicians will lay out the plan to attack this monster that has invaded your body or that of your loved one, and these dedicated, caring people are most certainly doing God's work. They will discuss the treatment, be it surgery, chemotherapy, radiation, seeds, rehab or otherwise. They will let you know the duration of the treatment, and the side effects that may come with the hoped-for cure. And to varying degrees, you or your loved one will fight this, because there is no choice. My hope is that you will fight it with everything you've got. Not everyone does.

I wrote this book to help you with the emotional aspects to this invisible fiend, and what this crisis might do to your everyday life. How it will affect your relationship with your spouse. What might happen at work. The difficulty you may have focusing, sleeping, and getting along with others. The financial havoc this disease brings down upon families, and the fallout that results.

Cancer can and will devour a relationship, unless you are armed with the knowledge to battle that insidious side of the disease. For with this diagnosis comes anger, fear, anxiety, despair, and loneliness. All of those emotions are normal. But trying to deal with them on your own can lead to depression and destructive behavior.

I hope that some day, cancer victims, cancer couples and cancer families will be given the tools—the professional help— to fight this aspect of a two-front war. But because so few have insurance for psychological help or family counseling, they receive the diagnosis and the plan for the physical attack on the disease, and then are sent to the parking lot, numb and afraid. Most have no idea how to break the news to the family, to colleagues at work, and to children. Sleep becomes difficult, or impossible. Your ability to concentrate at work wanes.

And if you are the husband of a wife with cancer, take heed. Learn that she needs far more than a chauffer to and from the hospital.

This is the story of what happened to my wife and me, from my perspective. I did not handle the emotional side of this disease well at all, and I paid a heavy price for it. I made a lot of mistakes you can easily avoid. I hope this story, and the lessons you glean from it, will help keep your relationship intact and help you learn how to interact with your loved one during this horrible time.

You can get through this. Your relationship can survive cancer after surviving cancer. If that sounds strange, you will soon understand what I mean.

Chapter 1

To this day, I can't say what it was that was so infuriating about the man—what it was exactly that made me explode. Was it his attitude of utter condescension? His pinched little smirk? Probably both – that and the tone of his voice when he said, "You had better bill some big hours over the next couple months."

In the time it took for my so-called colleague to say the words, the seething mixture of rage, fear, despair and frustration; the constant ache in my gut, the emotional bile, and all the other venoms that had been splashing around inside me for the previous ten months boiled over – and splattered all over his fine tailored suit.

Trembling with anger, I told him that, well then, if he wouldn't mind waiting, I'd run right home, fetch my brittle, radiation-burned wife and have her apologize to him for her cancer and the loss of income it had caused him. I'd put a wig on her head, wrap her in a coat and bring her straightaway to the downtown law office he and I shared, so that she could tell him personally just how sorry she was.

For a moment, he said nothing. Then, with a dismissive air, he mentioned that perhaps he had chosen his words poorly. This he followed with a smirk. Again with the smirk.

Believe me, I'm not a violent person. I'd seen enough of it growing up. But in this instance, there was no thinking about it. I went horizontal on the guy. I came down on him like a wolverine on amphetamines. I wanted to rip off his face and show it to him. If a sharp pencil had been handy, I would have jammed it into his eyes.

The two other attorneys in the room pulled me back and dragged me down the hall. A third joined us, and they took me to the elevator, pressed the button to the lobby and took me outside to Fountain Square, the focal point of Cincinnati's downtown.

There on the square, shaking from the after affects of the adrenalin that had surged through my body, I sobbed like a man who had lost everything.

I was out of money, out of hope and running on empty.

Chapter 2

My wife and I married in 1983. I was thirty and she was twenty seven. Our honeymoon lasted three years. In 1986, a cluster of lumps appeared in her neck. She underwent surgery to have them removed. For several days, we held our breath. Finally, the results came back from the lab. The doctor said the tests showed the lumps were benign. What a relief! We celebrated that night by going out to dinner at a fine restaurant.

No one ever questions good news. It's not human nature to question good news. We rejoice, trade high fives and celebrate for as long as it lasts. We don't bother to verify it. We just happily accept it as truth.

But when the news is bad, the questions start to fly. "Why me? How could you fire me? Why are you doing this to me, God? Who do I talk to about a second opinion?"

That's how it was with the results from those first biopsies. As much as it should be an instinctive reaction to ask for a second opinion on something so critical, I was all too ready to accept the verdict that the tumors were benign. We never thought about asking another pathologist to look at the slides. We dodged a bullet, so it seemed.

When my wife returned to have her stitches removed, she told the doctor we had decided to put off having children until her health questions were resolved. He dismissed her concerns with a wave of his hand, saying the lumps were probably the result of an allergic reaction to the bad Ohio Valley air, which follows the trough of the Ohio River and tends to just stay there and collect huge clouds of allergens. It's one of the reasons the Ohio Valley is thought to have an unusually high cancer rate.

Our first child was conceived two weeks later.

Every dad-to-be remembers the moment he learned he would become a father. All of the standard questions raced through my mind – except that they were anything but standard to me. Boy? Girl? Athlete? What would he or she look like or grow up to be? Would this baby be healthy and whole? Am I worthy of this gift from God? Many of my thoughts were focused on how fortunate we were to conceive, when so many couples today cannot.

We were so happy. The tumors were benign, and we were pregnant with our first child. Our joy completely blotted out the fear that had preceded it.

But then, two months into our pregnancy, another lump appeared in my wife's neck. I asked her to go to the doctor to get it checked out. She refused. She simply reminded me of what the doctor said. I relented, but got her to agree we would keep an eye on it.

By the fourth month, it had grown to nearly the size of a golf ball. I wore myself out trying to convince her to have it checked. She refused, saying the results would be the same as before. It would be a waste of time, she said.

That wasn't working for me. I made an appointment with a second physician without telling her. On the day of that appointment, I got her into the car on the premise of going out for an early dinner. When we pulled into the hospital parking lot, she was furious. At that point, I didn't care. I knew I was doing the right thing.

Three doctors examined her. They told us they were almost certain it was cancer. The location of the lumps was a clue. Her age was a clue. The fact the lumps had returned so quickly was another clue.

It was one tough night, the first of many. You pray, you bargain. You beg Him for no bad news. The next morning, my wife underwent a second procedure, this time without anesthesia, because you can't administer anesthesia to a pregnant woman and not expect consequences to the child. I tried hard in the waiting room not to think about what it must be like to have your neck sliced open while awake, enduring that pain out of concern for your unborn child.

This time, the results were back in a day. The diagnosis: Hodgkin's disease, a type of cancer also known as lymphoma, so called because it spreads from one lymph node group to another.

LOOKING BACK/LESSONS LEARNED

➤While it would not have made a difference in our case, not forcing the issue about my wife seeing a doctor would have been a mistake. Early detection means everything in the fight against cancer. You know that already, right? If not, get yourself and your loved one checked. Then stay on a regular schedule to get checked in the future.

➤Sometimes you have to take charge if a loved one is ignoring a lump, or simply sticking his or her head in the sand. Some people handle crises head on. Others try to ignore them. Still others fall apart. My way of dealing with my wife's unwillingness to see a doctor was not ideal. But you absolutely, positively have to keep talking. Say you love him/her, say you are worried. Say something like, "My darling, what would you do if it was me?" And if you're the one who is afflicted, think about the fact that your loved ones want to be in this fight with you. Let them in.

➤This type of conversation can take place during the illness, too. Many patients, toward the end of their radiation or chemotherapy treatment, decide that they have had enough. They are so sick and do not want any further treatment. It's best to follow the oncologist's advice. But let's face it—it is so tough to endure a treatment so draconian that, at times, it feels like the cure is worse than the disease. But it does save lives. Whatever you do, bring love into all your conversations. Doing so generates strength where you may have thought none was possible.

Chapter 3

We met in late 1980, at my workplace. She had a friend who worked there, and we were introduced. Our first date was about a week later. It was wonderful.

We came from humble beginnings. She had a large family— four siblings and parents who struggled financially. I had two younger brothers. My father was an angry and occasionally violent Irishman who never saw his high school graduation day. My mother was a wonderful but neurotic woman who lived in fear of her husband.

My childhood home was a tense place. Our dinners were eaten in total silence. My father worked nights, so when he left the house at 7:30, my mother, my brothers and I all breathed a sigh of relief. He had Tuesdays and Wednesdays off, so we never saw him much. He played golf from dawn to dusk on those days. Thus, the Murphy boys learned very early on that we had to fend for ourselves. It was tough going to little league baseball games without our dad ever being there. We missed all the father/son communion breakfasts and athletic dinners. It was an uphill climb trying to become a starter on any kind of team when you had no one to teach you the game.

I remember my father being very upset when I got cut from a select football team. I said nothing, but years later, I so very much related to Rocky Balboa when he said to his manager, "How can I be champ if I ain't got no locker, Mick?" In other words, how could I have been a football player if no one ever threw me a pass or taught me anything about the game?

Growing up, we all suffered differently. I kept it all inside, with one exception. I decided my junior year to flunk every class to get his attention. It didn't work. Instead, it kept me from gaining admission to a decent college. My brothers? Well, they raised some hell. They partied hard, and one got into a criminal scrape. The scars ran deep. After 18, we were pretty much on our own.

As for my new girlfriend, her growing up years had been mostly uneventful. But she had an old-fashioned father who thought post high school education for girls was a waste of money and time. She went to college anyway and excelled, but never finished.

Alcoholism had touched both of our families. Three of my four grandparents were alcoholics. My mother also abused alcohol, increasingly so after my father left her. The parents of the woman who became my wife at times drank too much by today's standards.

How you handle crisis in part depends on the values you shaped growing up. I was repeatedly exposed to my old man's expressions, of which he meant every word:

"When the going gets tough, the tough get going."
"If you want it done right, do it yourself."
"Quit complaining—nobody gives a damn anyway."

"Men do not cry. Only women and babies cry."

Before the diagnosis, my wife and I both worked. We saved to buy two decent cars to replace our beaters. We traveled to places like Bermuda and Germany. We had fun.

She was quiet by nature. I am Irish. No one would accuse me of being bashful. Even in those first three wonderful years, I had to sometimes struggle to learn what she was thinking. I wore my heart on my sleeve. For the most part, she kept her emotions to herself.

We loved each other. She supported and encouraged me while I finished law school. She helped me study for the bar exam by feeding me healthy meals and keeping me loose. She gave me a sense of purpose. She had a heart of gold.

But as I mentioned, she had a quiet, reserved nature. On several occasions when we would go out to dinner with friends, I would be asked the next day if she felt okay, or if something was wrong. I always explained it away – she was quiet, an observer. But her quietude also extended to me and made it difficult to break through to her feelings about so many things.

I imagine now that perhaps her quiet nature was a result of her voice not being heard at home growing up.

My sense is that both of us were raised to fend for ourselves. Asking for help was not something we were encouraged to do.

LOOKING BACK/LESSONS LEARNED

➤ How are you wired to handle crisis? We are all different. You have seen families like the Kennedys endure crisis after crisis, with dignity and strength. Think of Rose Kennedy, the matriarch, enduring the husband's death, then standing at the graves of her two sons, John and Robert, gunned down by maniacs. Conversely, we all know people who get a hangnail and fall to pieces. And then there is a third group—those who appear on the surface to be handling crisis well—but inside are suffering in quiet despair. That was me. Which describes you?

➤ When faced with a crisis like cancer, how you were raised will definitely have a bearing on how you cope. And if you were raised like me, told to "grin and bear it" while bleeding, you may be the most vulnerable to the emotional side of this disease–or for that matter, any life-altering hardship.

➤ If you are facing cancer, you need help, no matter how strong you think you are. Everybody facing cancer needs to weep. It is not a sign of weakness—it is a sign of normality! The human spirit is like a balloon—if you put too much air in it, it will blow. You cannot stifle these emotions. Tears are a remarkable release. It's okay to let them flow.

Chapter 4

My wife was home alone when the physician's assistant called with the pathology report.

"Your tumors are malignant Mrs. Murphy. Sorry. You should come in tomorrow at one o'clock."

Why couldn't that physician's assistant find a better way to break the news? Can anyone be that insensitive? My wife was hysterical when she called me at the office. I grabbed my keys, jumped into my car and ran every red light and stop sign on the way home.

My mind was racing as well. Could this be a mistake? Only five months earlier, we were told the lumps were harmless! Why did the physician's assistant call her, when I'd left clear instructions with the doctor's office to call me? How could she be so callous?

I remember clutching the steering wheel with a death grip. My chest felt as if steel bands were constricting around me. I could barely breathe. And I remember searching for words. What would I say to my wife when I got home?

I found her on the kitchen floor with the phone still off the hook. She hadn't moved after calling me. That emotional scar will never heal. Seeing her like that—this beautiful pregnant mother to be, crumpled on the floor—there are no words. Healthcare professionals, take heed.

The next day, we were at Christ Hospital in Cincinnati. It's quite a sobering experience to walk into a hospital wing and see a sign that reads "ONCOLOGY" and know you're not just passing through. Once again, my chest tightened. I can't imagine what she felt. We didn't talk about it. We didn't know how.

We were there all day. During a private moment, the doctors told me of two procedures for determining how far advanced the cancer was. They referred to it as staging the disease. Once they knew how far along the cancer had progressed, they could begin to determine the best options for fighting it.

One procedure involved injecting dye into her bloodstream, then taking pictures of her lymph nodes. Problem was, the dye would be a fatal injection of poison to our baby. The second procedure was called a laparotomy, where an incision is made from the rib cage to the pelvis. With the patient opened down the middle, surgeons physically examine the organs, starting with the spleen. That surgery also would kill our baby.

But if the doctors couldn't immediately determine how far the disease had spread, they wouldn't know how to treat it. Nor would they have any idea of her chances of survival, or whether she would even make it through the remaining five months of her pregnancy. The oncologist told me point blank that he and his team had never faced this dilemma, with two lives at stake. He simply didn't know what to do. I was grateful for his honesty. He asked us to consider going to Stanford University Hospital, the Mecca for Hodgkin's disease treatment, research and care. I would have gone to Afghanistan if it was the best place to go.

They took bone marrow that day. That caused her agonizing pain. I spent the time in the waiting area in somewhat of a trance.

It was all happening so quickly. Just days earlier, we were a normal happy couple, excited and swept up with joy at the prospect of having our first child and presenting our parents with a grandchild. We had started to talk about names. Now, I was sitting in a cold room with year-old magazines, wondering if both lives would make it. I wondered if I would ever see my child's face. And I grieved for my beautiful bride, for I knew what that baby meant to her. She was just so happy and content. And now this … how could this happen to us?

The oncologist arranged an appointment for us at Stanford University Hospital for 10 days hence. He told me to come back in seven days so he could give me the results from the previous procedures to take to Stanford. He shook my hand, and told me to hang in there.

And then my wife and I were walking to the parking lot, numb and in silence.

LOOKING BACK/LESSONS LEARNED

➢There is no answer to the question why. I asked that question *for years*, and the only purpose it served was to intensify my pain. You will think about all the jerks you know who seem to live happy, stress free lives, and you ask yourself, *why did this happen to us?* Trust me—the earlier you can come to grips with the fact that there is no answer to the question why, the better off you will be.

➢God did not do this to you. For a long time, I asked Him why. Sometimes I threw a fist up in the air. What did I do and what did we do to deserve this? Years later, I learned—we had done nothing to deserve this. I resigned myself to learning the answer to this and many other questions when I pass to the next world, which I believe will be one of peace, love and pain free. Cancer or any debilitating disease is a bad break. It is so unfair. But if it rang your doorbell as it did ours, do not waste one minute blaming God. Instead, ask Him to give you His strength to get through it.

➢If you are at this early stage where you have just learned the dreaded news, try to find a support group. Attend a meeting and introduce yourself to others who have walked down the road you are about to travel. Sure, if you are anything like me, the last thing you want to do is break down in front of a bunch of strangers. But you will be amazed at how much someone in the same predicament can help and support you. If you are unable to discuss your feelings to a group, then talk to your pastor, your priest, your rabbi. If you have insurance coverage or the financial wherewithal, now is the time to seek professional counseling from a psychologist or a psychiatrist. Looking back, I wish I had done that. I wish we both would have had a preview to the emotional movie we were about to experience – separately as well as together. More the former than the latter, as it turned out.

➢ Most hospitals and cancer clinics, with the help of mental health professionals, have developed a protocol on how best to break the news to a human being that he or she has cancer. Telephoning a pregnant woman home alone, to inform her that she has cancer, is cruel. I can still remember my wife's body crumpled on our kitchen floor. It's an image I will never be completely free of. Fortunately, what happened to my wife rarely if ever occurs.

➢ If you have just recently received the bad news, understand that emotions will run high. That is normal. Other than following the advice of your doctors and seeking emotional help, make no major decisions until things calm down.

Chapter 5

So home we went – a short 20-minute drive across the Ohio River. The bone marrow procedure left her sore and aching. She was bothered more about being put into an MRI machine, a then relatively new invention, knowing that no real data existed as to the potential harm this device could have on our growing baby.

I struggled to find the words to ease her fear, but they wouldn't come to me. It was all I could do to drive home. My heart was beating so fast with what I assumed was an anxiety attack. It would be the first of many to come.

We walked into the house, and she went directly to bed. What had been a beautiful, joyful mother-to-be 48 hours earlier was now a woman consumed with grief, uncertainty, and fear. While she rested, I answered the gut-wrenching phone calls from her parents and siblings and broke the news to her friends. No one prepares you for this sort of thing. Some I spoke with cried, and I didn't know how to respond. Others asked question after question, for which I had little or no answers. Mostly, I remember the tightness in my chest and the dull, relentless ache in my head.

We spent the next several days in relative silence, too focused on our own emotions to do much talking. The joy of her pregnancy was gone. She spent most of those days just sitting there with her hand on her belly, as if to reassure herself that at least for the moment, the baby was fine.

For me, the nights leading to the trip to Stanford were the worst. Over and over I asked why? Why her, the kindest most gentle soul I knew? Why not me? Why during our first pregnancy? Why did this monster choose to attack us? I know now that there are no answers to these questions, but I didn't then. All I knew was that we were alone. When the doctors at Christ sent us home, they sent us home alone. We were unequipped to deal with this nightmare.

Both of us believed in God, but we were not frequent churchgoers. I talked to God often, but never much beneath the surface. I had no family nearby for support. She had plenty of family members around, but they were having as much difficulty dealing with the situation as we were. It was too much for them to bear. Her dad was devastated. He could hardly speak. But they were there for her.

The stress symptoms had already started. It began with sleepless nights and headaches. My stomach went sour, and there were days when I was in the bathroom five or six times a day. And that was just in the first week.

I believe the very worst fear is fear of the unknown. The wait to get to Stanford for answers was unbearable. And with anything that has to be biopsied, the wait between not knowing and knowing can be days or weeks, through no fault of the healthcare professionals.

For instance, a CAT Scan I had a few years ago showed what the radiologist thought was a tumor. I received the news of that by telephone, because the doctor's office had to schedule a follow-up appointment. That appointment was five days after the telephone call. What do you think was going through my mind in those five days? That this was no big deal? That I was going to be fine? I tried saying that. But of course, the pessimistic side of that tug of war was by far the stronger. I kept thinking the worst. Is it basic human nature to do that? I have come to learn that the stronger your faith is in God, coupled with a good circle of family and friends, the more likely you are to have a positive outlook in these types of matters.

In times like these, my tendency was to retreat. To stay away from people so I didn't have to talk about it. I went to a very dark place inside of me, and that is the very worst thing you can do.

LOOKING BACK/LESSONS LEARNED

➤ If I could go back in time, I would have sought some help at the outset. I realize now I needed someone to tell me that what I was feeling and thinking was normal. Someone to make me understand grief, and help show me how to cope with stress. I will repeat this several times—I strongly recommend that if you are in the throes of this disease, find your pastor, a therapist, or a support group as soon as possible. As you read on, you will understand more fully why. Me? I thought I could handle it. I was a former union truck driver in New York City. A former fireman who was a good street fighter back in the day. I can handle this, I thought. *When the going gets tough...*

➤ Note that it did not take long for me to suffer from anxiety, with a fast heartbeat, a tight chest, and stomach distress. Yep, this situation started breaking me down in short order. I was experiencing very real physical issues. My problem was what I said earlier—the tough guy stubbornness—coupled with no support system. So be smarter than me. From the very beginning, seek out people who can help you. There is truly strength in numbers, and comfort in knowing you are not alone.

➤ I had such a hard time calling her parents, siblings, and friends. Call after call, the knot in my chest grew tighter. I kept thinking—this person asked me to call after we got out of the hospital—but what do I tell them? And regardless of how I say it, what I have to tell them is going to make them very upset. Sure, the calls had to be made. But I should have used that opportunity to ask them for help. It would have made us both feel better.

➤This is a two-sided disease. It attacks the cancer victim physically, and the entire family emotionally, from day one. The medical profession helps you fight the physical side, but who will help you fight on the emotional front?

Chapter 6

On the following Friday, the slides from my wife's first surgery failed to arrive at the oncologist's office as requested. I immediately suspected the pathologist at the first hospital had gone into damage control mode. He must have misread the slides. The oncologist knew it too.

He asked me to step outside his office while he called the pathologist at the first hospital. At one point in the conversation, I heard him yell, "There are two lives to consider, not one! How can I send these two kids to Stanford without those slides? They have a right to know!"

It was the first of several episodes when anger boiled inside me. I finally got my hands on the missing slides after threatening not only to go to the newspaper, but to inflict bodily harm to anyone foolish enough to get in my way.

It's a sad fact of life: There are those among us completely devoid of conscience. The individuals at the first hospital who decided not to turn over the slides could have cared less if a woman and her child lived or died. They were more concerned with covering their own mistakes and willing to jeopardize two lives to do so.

I knew in my gut that my wife had been misdiagnosed the first time, and it ate at me badly. By trying to prevent us from getting the slides and frozen tumor slices, it was clear someone had made an unfortunate but serious mistake. The dilemma that resulted was about to force my wife to make a life-and-death decision. Who was that mystery person, I wondered? How did this happen? These questions in reality were doing nothing but making me seethe. Anger is useless but very dangerous, and mine started early in this process.

I spent numerous nights leading up to our visit phoning doctors I knew to try to learn as much as I could about Stanford. I also had friends call. It all came back 100 percent positive. Stanford had a reputation for being the very best institution in the world for this particular type of cancer. Having strong suspicions that we were victimized with incorrect news from the first surgery, it gave me a measure of relief knowing we would be in the best hands possible. I wanted nothing less for my wife. I wanted to do anything I could to tilt the odds in her favor. Most of all, I wanted her to see the child that was growing inside her, the child she loved more than her own life.

Yet at no time did I consider finding the best person to help us emotionally. It never crossed my mind.

Work was tough. I told my assistant the terrible news, but overall tried to keep it quiet. Since I did not have all the answers to the myriad of questions I knew would come, I was not up to answering the same questions from 60 or 70 people. I was already fatigued from the worry and the sleep deprivation it caused. Concentrating was very difficult, and at times impossible.

The 10 days until our departure to Stanford ticked by slowly. We tried to carry on as if our lives hadn't been turned upside-down. Each night, we struggled to find conversation.

We were avoiding the elephant in the room. How far advanced is the cancer? Was she misdiagnosed? How long has she had cancer? Will she make it? What is to become of this child inside her? What would we do if the doctors at Stanford told us our best option was to abort? Who can make that decision? If you can believe it, we did not discuss any of these questions. I knew she had to be thinking about them, just like me. But silence entered our home, right on the heels of the cancer.

Finally, we were on the flight to California. At around 30,000 feet, my wife brought up the abortion question. She told me she had decided to put our child's life before her own. She would leave it in God's hands. That conversation, in hushed tones, brought tears to us both. We were still numb from the previous 10 days. We were flying into the unknown, very possibly to receive even more devastating news. A flight attendant asked us if everything was okay. I smiled weakly and said yes. The fact that we were not the normal happy pregnant couple must have been evident.

That night in our hotel room, the mind racing continued. I was scared. Being somewhat small and thin, my wife was showing. It made the other life involved very, very real for me. I just had to look at her to see the baby. This was not a fetus—this was our child.

From the moment she told me the glorious news that we were pregnant, I had visions in my mind's eye of this baby. Of holding my firstborn in my arms, seeing her face for the first time. And here we were, in a strange room in a strange land, wondering what the next day would bring.

Try as I might to do otherwise, I had only dark thoughts of her not making it, or losing both of them. I thought of losing the child, and what that would do to her psyche, as she faced an uphill cancer fight. I thought about raising a child without her mother. Of having to someday down the road explain to that child what her wonderful mother was like. Could I raise a child by myself? Who would help me?

I tried so hard to silence these thoughts, to no avail. It was a long night.

LOOKING BACK/LESSONS LEARNED

➤Talking about the cancer, the struggle, answering the questions—it's one painful experience, one trauma after another. But avoiding it is worse. People want to know because they care. They want to help, even if all they can do is pray or light a candle. Talking to your loved ones is even more important. Silence indeed invaded our home. It was overwhelming. I did not know what to say or how to comfort her. In retrospect, I wish we would have dedicated a chunk of time every day putting our feelings into words and sharing those words with each other.

➤Prior to this horrible event, I had never truly lost my temper. Yes, I was in my fair share of fistfights as a kid, but I never started them. But it took no time at all for me to be filled with rage at those folks who wouldn't produce the slides from the first surgery. I was shocked at how strong that emotion was. I truly wanted to physically hurt somebody. But that wasn't me. It was as if I had become another person. Anger is like pain—it is a signal that something is wrong with you. You have to deal with it to keep it from boiling over and coming to the surface in ways you are sure to regret. How? Again—get with a mental health professional, or your pastor/spiritual advisor. Get with a doctor, or a support group. Don't let anger destroy you. It will if you let it.

➤If you are the one that has the cancer, you can already see the incredible pain on the faces of your family. The news hits them just as hard. The disease afflicts them as well, in ways that are different but no less profound. You can fight the disease, but your spouse, your partner and your family members cannot. And that is an immense source of frustration for them. They will not be in the radiation machine. They will not be enduring the chemo. They will be in the waiting room pacing, praying, crying, or home waiting on a phone call. So let them in! Start talking about your feelings, so they can better understand you, and then urge them to talk. That macho husband of yours, or brother or friend, may be putting on a nice strong mask, but in reality he is hurting. It is a very different dynamic being the non-cancer "other," but it is almost as difficult, because they want to take this from you. They want to be taking the chemo in your place. They would rather be the one vomiting in the back of the car on the ride home from the treatments. It's what love is all about. And love is what this life is all about, so let it flow.

➤ No doubt you already understand that I was struggling with demons I could not control. Mental health professionals are forever telling their patients to separate the things that they can control from what they cannot. You are told to visualize taking the things you cannot control and putting them in a closet and locking the door. If you cannot control it, stop worrying about it. It is hard to do, but it is excellent advice!

➤ What can you control? Trying to make life easier for your loved one. Maintaining your own mental and physical health so that you can be a good helper to the person going through this harrowing journey. You can take care of things around the house or perform other tasks to ease the burden. And you can pray.

Chapter 7

Dawn arrived, and with a combination of dread and anticipation, we followed the directions that led us to Stanford University Hospital. The place is huge. I remember asking at the information desk where we had to go, and walking down long hallways toward Oncology. My heart was pounding and once again, there was the now-familiar tightness in my chest. She remained as she had for the last previous 10 days—very quiet.

After filling out what seemed like endless reams of paperwork, we were put into a small room. We did not have to wait long. The door opened, and I remember being instantly comforted by a warm greeting from a team of "grey hairs." We hadn't realized that Stanford is a teaching institution, and the physician teachers saw my wife's case as a valuable opportunity to learn. Pregnant cancer patients, they told us, are rare.

After outlining for us what would take place that day, they excused themselves to look at the materials we brought with us – in particular, the slides and tumor tissue from the first surgery. When they returned, my fear became a reality.

Their review of the slides from the first and second surgeries confirmed that the first pathologist had misread the slides. So much for having early detection working for us. My wife had cancer for over a year.

The Stanford doctors also had no way of knowing how far the cancer had advanced because, as we had been told at Christ Hospital in Cincinnati, they couldn't do the dye exam or the laparotomy, the two procedures that would have told us all how far the disease had progressed.

The doctors told us what they knew, what they didn't and what they wished they did. They explained the risks of carrying the child full term, particularly since the cancer had a significant head start. When they finished, my wife told them she could not picture herself at the age of 70 sitting on a porch at sunset, wondering if she could have saved this child. She would rather be dead.

A long silent moment followed. I looked at their faces, fully expecting that they would urge her to abort. After all, we were on the left coast, geographically and politically. But what I saw in that frozen moment of silence were a whole bunch of moist eyes. Then Dr. Steve Hancock, Stanford's chief of radiation therapy, lit up the room.

"Great!" he said. "Then we'll save you and your baby."

I can't begin to tell you how it felt to hear those words and the optimism behind them. Dr. Hancock would see us through the entire experience. Note to all docs: Hope is a powerful force. It's what Dr. Hancock gave us. He exuded confidence. He made me believe, at least for the moment, we would be okay. He also energized the whole team. We had our mission statement. I decided right then – this is where she was going to be treated, even if I had to rob a bank to make it happen.

Sure, there are cases where it's not realistic to be so hopeful, times when a patient is in the late stages of cancer when it's first discovered. No one wants to be misled. But I know for sure that if you give up hope, you don't stand much of a chance. And miracles do happen. Doctors see them all the time.

It was a long, stressful day. We learned a lot about Hodgkin's disease, how it spreads and where it attacks. And we learned how it is treated, normally. We were informed of the various specialties and departments that would be involved, including radiation therapy, oncology, X-rays/radiology and surgery. We learned how long the treatment would take, survival rates and the side effects of the treatment. We also learned the risks, especially the risk of delaying treatment. I understood why they had to tell us, in spite of everyone's universal desire to save our child. I knew exactly what they were saying.

The doctor set an initial goal of carrying our developing baby into the seventh month. They wanted us to fly to California every 30 days so she could have chest x-rays done. She was not thrilled about this, worried as she was about the effects on the baby, but they told her she had no choice. Once the cancer spread to her chest, treatment had to begin. It had already spread to the other side of her neck, which caused the doctors to reclassify it from stage one to stage two. This disease is a progressive one, the doctors told us, and the next logical place for it to spread would be her chest.

When the day ended, we made our appointment for thirty days hence, said our thanks and waved goodbye. Once again, we walked to a parking lot, got into our rented car, and made our way to the airport, with our individual thoughts and fears.

We had a roadmap to get through the pregnancy and for what it would take to beat the cancer. But as we headed to the airport to fly back to Kentucky, we had no plan for dealing with our emotions. We were going home not knowing how far advanced the cancer was. We didn't know if she would make it through the pregnancy or even to the next Stanford visit in 30 days. Other questions were racing through my mind. Would the bank let us slide on our mortgage payments? Would the car loan company give a damn about us or would we lose our car? If she made it, how would we cope with the loss of her income for a year or more? If the baby survives, three mouths to feed!

All of these questions rattled in my brain on the plane ride home while my wife slept. She was exhausted physically and emotionally. I was, too. But my body wasn't fighting an invader like hers was. And the questions, barking at me like angry dogs, would not let me rest.

LOOKING BACK/LESSONS LEARNED

➤Finding the right medical team is key for a variety of reasons. Obviously, the doctors have to know what they are doing. So check them out, which is much easier to do today than when my wife and I were going through it— just turn on your computer. Also, ask your family doctor for several recommendations. It is so important for you to be comfortable with the medical team. It is even more important that you believe they care about you. The two Cs are essential to me—confidence and compassion.

➤If you have insurance, get someone on the phone who can tell you what doctors/hospitals are covered and which ones are "out of network" or not covered. Hopefully, your situation is not as complicated as ours was, but if you have a rare condition, you can battle for coverage. For instance, large healthcare companies will allow you to travel out of state if the doctor/hospital are "in network" in that state. Call and request a personal representative— and ask. You will never get what you do not ask for. Which in turn means you need to know *what* to ask for. Knowledge is power.

➤Knowledge is also power when it comes to learning about the disease and the plan for the cure. The very worst thing you can do is to stick your head in the sand, even though what you're experiencing is certainly overwhelming. Knowledge is also important because you can help the doctors assess the progress being made, so they know that if plan A is not working, it is time for plan B.

➤ Knowing the details can also help you and your loved ones plan. For instance, if you will be undergoing chemotherapy, which weeks will be the worst? You can figure out what days to ask off from work or plan to ask for additional help from family or friends.

➤ Knowing yourself is important, too. Is it time to talk to someone to go unload your burden? To stay strong? To deal with the terrible stress and anxiety? Say yes, especially if you are a man. Women usually bring in their family and friends into their world when times are difficult. Men often do not. That is the wrong move. Cancer is a formidable foe, so get the help you need. Or suffer needlessly like I did.

Chapter 8

When we were newlyweds, my wife and I lived in a small apartment in Louisville, Kentucky. I worked for a large law firm. She worked for a major airline. Little did we know how lucky we were that she had a job with an employer that would bend the rules and permit us to fly free back and forth to California, even when she was sick and unable to work.

It was only a matter of weeks after our honeymoon when she started hinting rather strongly that she would like to move back to Northern Kentucky. We met there, and that is where her family lived. I got a kick out of that. She never said a word about moving back home when we were dating! But I knew she was close to her parents and her four brothers and sisters, and she missed her Northern Kentucky friends.

So I agreed to the move, even though I enjoyed my job and my colleagues immensely. I quickly found a job with a law firm in Cincinnati, so we moved back six months after we married. In one way, this move was a blessing, because we would later receive a great deal of help, love and support from her wonderful family in our time of need. But the down side was to come in the form of my new Cincinnati employer, who saw employees as faceless, nameless profit centers.

I had two brothers. One lived far away in North Carolina, the other followed me to Kentucky. My parents were divorced. My mother lived in Pennsylvania, and was incapable of helping due to her drinking problem. My father? He lived in Florida and for long periods, we did not speak. So unlike my wife, I did not have a family support system. I didn't think I needed one.

We bought our first house when we returned to Northern Kentucky. It was a market home. We were thrilled to have a brand new, 1,800-square-foot house with a two-car garage, our own little slice of heaven. The two of us were making about the same amount of money, with a mortgage, car payments and my student loans taking a good portion of our paychecks.

Neither of us came into the marriage with any money. We had a modest wedding, with a reception in the back yard of her parents' home. I came into the marriage with no assets other than an old car. So when the cancer came, the financial aspect of the disease was yet another thing we were unprepared for. Our parents could not help with money, nor could our respective siblings.

On the plane ride home, I started to think about how we could get her treated at Stanford. Would our health insurance cover her out of state? How much would a house cost to rent for five months? Who could come out there and help us with our child? I knew the baby would have to be with her.

We certainly didn't have the money to move to California. But after meeting that wonderfully talented and upbeat medical team, I knew they would give her the best chance to live, so I had to figure out a way. She was putting her life on the line to save our child. She deserved the best. Plus, the physicians at the best hospital in Cincinnati had sent us there, because they didn't have the answers.

As it turned out, our insurance would cover most but not all of our medical bills. But the reality was that our percentage of the medical bills from a hospital that our carrier said was "out of network" was beyond what we could afford.

We had four and a half months to go full term, and about two and a half months to give the child a fighting chance. The first job I had back home was to again convey to family and friends that the cancer had advanced to stage 2 at least. I had to let everyone know we were still flying blind because of the inability to determine conclusively if the cancer was stage 3 or 4, because the tests that would normally be done to make that determination would kill the child. I had to explain that our doctors thought they could get us to the seventh month and give the baby a shot at life, but that they had no real knowledge of whether pregnancy slows or quickens the speed of Hodgkin's disease. And finally, I would let everyone know we met a bunch of talented, caring and dedicated physicians and staff who *wanted* us to be treated there.

I had to figure out how to muster enough money to get her treated at Stanford. I made $750.00 a week before taxes. Her pay was about $600.00 a week, but it was about to change soon due to maternity leave. Our car payments were around $350.00. Our mortgage was more than $900.00 a month. Taxes, insurance, student loans, food, baby clothes … you get the picture. I called a few realtors in Palo Alto to find out what it would cost to rent a small house near the hospital, and was stunned to hear the numbers – $3,000 or more per month for a 1,200-square-foot two-bedroom bungalow.

Then there was the issue of caring for the baby. How could we do that? Leave her at home with her grandmother? No way that could happen – mom needed to be with her newborn. But flying out babysitters? We certainly could not afford that. But how do you ask someone to spend hundreds of dollars on a round-trip ticket to San Francisco and use one of two vacation weeks to tend to a newborn and her sick mom?

Here is the point – sometimes this disease will totally overwhelm you, if you let it. You will feel that you are in a 20-foot hole with no ladder to get out. Cancer comes at you in so many ways. Financially, I could not afford to get my wife the best care. It ate me up day after day, trying to figure out how to rob Peter to pay Paul. If she did not go to Stanford and wound up dying, I would spend the rest of my life wondering if she would have made it. And I might someday have to look her child in the eye and explain it.

I did some smart things on the financial front but failed to do what I clearly needed to do. First, the smart things—I went to the bank that held our mortgage and told a vice president about our circumstances. I explained that in order to rent a home in California, we would have to forego our mortgage payments for six or seven months. He said fine, and wished me luck. I tried doing the same thing with the car loan company, although I never got a definite yes. I tried to figure out how we could cut expenses.

There was just so much to do.

LOOKING BACK/LESSONS LEARNED

➤What I did not do is ask anyone for financial help. Why? I have attended in my lifetime countless benefits for cancer families, kids with childhood illnesses whose parents were struggling, on and on and on. I had no problem contributing – I always did so, willingly and gladly. So why couldn't I ask someone to do that for us? I knew we could muster enough money to pay the rent in California for one, maybe two months or three months – but that was it. Still, four months out, I was…banking on money to fall out of the sky? Was it my pride? Was it because I thought asking for help meant I was weak? Maybe. Probably. Was it a part of my upbringing? No doubt about that.

➤And herein lies the big problem: Neither of us wanted to be a burden, not on each other, not on anybody. So we didn't ask. Was there help available for us financially had we looked? I am sure of it. Financial pressure is deadly on a marriage. It is one of the leading factors that cause divorce in a "normal" marriage, absent cancer or other crisis. Going broke ate at me. It made me feel like a failure.

➤Had I asked for financial help from my friends, I would have received it. Sure, some people would have said no. But the bottom line is, people want to help. It makes them feel good! It makes them feel they're part of the healing. What good is love if you can't show it? I saw my church raise $50,000 in a weekend for the Haiti earthquake in early 2010—for perfect strangers. Therein lies the riddle for me. I love to help people. I love the feeling I get when I can help relieve the pain of another human being. And yet, I could not ask for a dime. The result? Horrible stress and anxiety, which turned to anger and despair. A dangerous mix of emotions.

➤I am reminded of Christ's walk up the hill to Golgotha, where He was crucified. Three times He fell while carrying his cross. Each time, He accepted help from someone in the crowd. He allowed all three men to help carry that cross. I now understand the lesson Christ was teaching, even as He was approaching His crucifixion. It is okay to ask for help! Allow others to help you so they can get that wonderful feeling of lending a hand. Accept help. We all need it sooner or later. And whatever help you receive, there is so much joy in giving it right back when your friend is in need. One of my biggest mistakes in this process was my inability to ask for help. I could not admit that I was overwhelmed. Please do not make that mistake. Pride is one of the seven deadly sins, for good reason.

➤Men especially need to realize that it is okay to seek help. It is *not* a sign of weakness—it is a sign of strength, and smarts. I was not coping well at this juncture. I was eating antacids like they were candy, and smoking heavily. My stomach was killing me. And it would get worse, because I was trying to go it alone.

Chapter 9

So now the countdown began toward our child's viability. Each day was an eternity. We were fighting an enemy we could not see, and were powerless against. Each night, I felt as if the cancer had advanced another day. I felt helpless against it. And for a type A personality, that is not good.

Was it spreading? Would she make it? Physically? Emotionally? She began having nightmares. I woke up many times in the wee hours of the morning to find her downstairs on the couch, eaten up with the forces that had taken over her body.

I was going to work each day, but struggling with my workload. It was hard to focus. The word got out slowly but surely to everyone at the firm, and I received some words of encouragement. But no one offered to help carry my caseload, and no one sat me down to talk about tomorrow and the days after that.

As the days ticked by, we became like so many other couples forced to deal with cancer—totally unequipped to handle the tidal wave of fear, anger, dread, the whole weird tangle of emotions washing over us. My constant prayer for any other couple going through this is that they seek help, someone to guide them through the Byzantine maze of feelings that accompany any life-threatening disease.

Through it all, we tried to carry on as if nothing was out of the ordinary, each of us lost in our thoughts. It hurt knowing this was an enemy that I could not fight. She didn't want to be a burden on me, and I didn't want to express any fear at all to her. I wanted to be strong for her. I wanted to be her rock. I did not tell her I was vomiting or having serious emotional distress. I did not tell her I was falling behind at work. And as I look back, I believe she somehow decided that what was happening was her fault. That our wonderful marriage and the joy of pregnancy was gone because of what *she* had. That this disease was inside *her*, ergo she was the reason for the sorrow, despair and worry we were going through.

From a distance it seems so ridiculous. I looked at her each day—my beautiful pregnant wife—and loved her more for her decision to fight for our baby. Her courage overwhelmed me. But at the same time, she was worried sick that she had put so much pressure on me.

We made some other moves that, without meaning to, made things worse. For one thing, to save money, we stopped going out to dinner. We should not have done that. One of my favorite authors, Leo Buscaglia, tells a story about his immigrant Italian parents. His dad came home from work in the early afternoon one day and tearfully told the family he had been laid off. That night, his mother prepared an absolute feast, something like five courses. It was her way of conveying to her family that everything was going to be just fine. And she was right—Leo's dad got a better paying job a few weeks later. If he hadn't been laid off, he would never have found that better job. One door had to close before the other could open.

My wife and I sort of hunkered down, as if to keep our misery to ourselves. Being out, running into people we knew was difficult, because we were doing all we could do to stay composed. At the same time, we were both consumed with dark thoughts. What would become of our child? Would he or she survive? Would our child have birth defects because of the monthly X-rays?

And how my wife dreaded those monthly flights to Stanford leading up to the delivery date! She was so afraid the doctors would want to take her baby early. Her primary concern was her child, far beyond her own health. I could see what it was doing to her. It hurt knowing she wasn't sharing her pain with me. But I was doing the same to her, keeping everything inside.

LOOKING BACK/LESSONS LEARNED

➤ Does any of this sound familiar? If it does, then start talking. And don't stop talking until it all comes out! Communication is critical during any crisis. When internalized fear becomes verbal, its power is lessened. I wish I would have opened my mouth and said something like, "I am scared. I can't lose you. Will you fight? How can I help you? What can I do? What are you thinking?"

➤ The cancer is not your fault! Anger, fear, anxiety—they are all normal emotions. But you have to deal with them, not swallow them. You have to vomit them up and out. You have to be able to rely on others to keep those emotions from destroying you and your relationship. If you are fortunate enough to have insurance that covers psychological services, by all means get counseling. Go early before the emotions turn into ulcers.

➤ What was I doing during this time? Seething about the pathologist who had missed the cancer from the initial surgery—the man who put us in this position. I was angry at him, more than I knew. As I lay awake in bed at night, I wondered how I could afford a house in Palo Alto so my wife could have the best treatment possible. I wondered who would care for our baby for five to six months. I promised to be strong for her. No tears, no outward signs of worry or fear, at least not in her presence. But in reality, I was breaking down. I could not get the possibility of losing her and our baby out of my mind. I was constantly sick to my stomach.

➢ Think about it. Could any man handle all this alone? What *was* I thinking? I tried. I failed. I look back now, and it is hard to comprehend how foolish I was. I presumed that because no one at work seemed to care, no one at the first hospital where the cancer had been misdiagnosed cared, it meant no one cared. I presumed I would have to go it alone, just like I had all along.

➢ I did not have the tools for coping. I needed guidance. I needed someone to listen, to shepherd me from the wolves of terror and grief. Where do you turn when you are the one who has to be strong? I felt like a first time high wire acrobat, putting one foot in front of the other, hoping to God I would not fall. But there is no science to dealing with tragedy. You call on your faith, your strength, but no one can prepare you. Crisis comes to every life, always by surprise, always by ambush. It eats into your life in ways you can never imagine. I was walking through darkness, and I was walking alone. It didn't have to be that way. It doesn't have to be that way for you.

➢ Make a plan for taking care of yourself emotionally. Discuss it with your loved ones. Ask them to help you stick to it—to hold you accountable. You will not regret it.

Chapter 10

Youth is wasted on the young. Have you heard that before? It's true. Of course, I have the benefit of hindsight, recounting my mistakes nearly a quarter of a century after making them.

I've mentioned before that the thought of going broke ate away at me. I had to laugh once when a client who was a multi-millionaire many times over told me about how having all that money filled him with fear at the prospect of losing it. Ha! How I would have loved to be plagued with that obsession.

The fear of going broke is multiplied ten fold when you have been broke before. I spent my entire twenties broke. After graduating from college with a teaching degree, I was still struggling. The only teaching job I could find paid $7,800 a year. I had to drive a truck three or four nights a week to pay for my apartment, bills and student loans. When I left New York at age twenty-five to go to law school in Kentucky, I had enough money for less than one year. I was forced to sell my car to pay for tuition and books.

Think about it. How do you go on a date without a car? I had to rely on friends for rides, or take public transportation. It was as if I was back in high school! I was riding the bus again, to a place with a ton of students who had Roman numerals at the end of their names, with fancy cars and nice clothes.

What did this generate inside me? Humiliation, embarrassment, and shame. And a sense of isolation.

Was I justified in feeling this way? I was trying to achieve something great. I had the courage to leave home to pursue a law degree, building my own version of the American dream. I left my friends and two jobs to chase my dream, knowing I did not have the money for the full three years. And I made it! Instead of being embarrassed and humiliated, I should have been proud of the gumption and determination I showed during that three-year struggle.

This is definitely a man thing. We think money is a sign of success. Just look at the car commercials. The guy with the Lexus or Mercedes always gets the hot babes. You don't see any bombshell cuddling up next to the guy behind the wheel in Volkswagon ads.

Men tend to equate being broke to being a failure. I remember when my father was on strike for 126 days. My parents were taking my paper route money to help pay for groceries. I watched him constantly fretting and getting angrier by the day. And when my mother offered to look for work—wow. He blew up. What would the neighbors think? Luke Murphy not providing for his family? No way. He would not tolerate that. So instead, we ate cereal or scrambled eggs for dinner.

When my graduation day came, I clutched that precious law degree and told myself that my days of eating macaroni and cheese out of a box were in the rearview mirror. I was on my way out of poverty, walking into a new world of prosperity, where I would never worry about money again. Or so I thought.

I've seen lawyers in big firms fight over who gets the corner office because having the corner office is like having a badge that says "Big shot."

Perception becomes reality. So, during the four and a half months of waiting between the cancer diagnosis and the birth of our child, on top of the worry about my wife and the baby, I had far too much time to contemplate going broke again. I had too much time to think about my childhood dining room table, worried about annoying my dad, who felt like a little man because he had no money to buy us meat for dinner.

My father could not and would not ask for help. I remembered that. And the apple did not fall far from the tree.

LOOKING BACK/LESSONS LEARNED

➤The great John Wayne once said, "Life is tough, pilgrim. But it's even tougher if you're stupid." Back then, I fell into that category. Please don't be stupid!

➤Cancer tapped my wife and me on the shoulder. It wasn't my fault, and it wasn't her fault. If it has hit your house or extended family, no fault there either. You may be thinking, "Yes, but isn't that obvious?" It sounds so logical, so common sense to say it – but when the disease is swirling around you, invading every pocket of your life, and when you're going it alone, despite all logic, you do begin to look for places to lay the blame. Do not do that. Instead, find someone on the outside who will remind you of that.

➤Here is what I should have done. I should have asked my friends to loan me money. Many would have. It would have taken a ton of pressure off. And I would have paid them back. Every once in awhile, my wife would say we couldn't afford to be going to Stanford. And I would tell her to let me worry about that. It would have been such a relief to her if I could have told her I already had most of the money for the rent in Palo Alto, and the airfare for friends and family to help with the baby. I hope you can see that my pride caused her to worry more.

Chapter 11

Work became more difficult by the day. As noted earlier, the word that my wife had cancer had gotten around at the law firm where I worked. But as I stated, there was no effort on the part of the bosses to lighten my caseload. They dwell among us—people who care only about themselves.

It was at work during those 130 days leading up to the birth of our child that I learned many people cannot face you when they know you are in the midst of a crisis. They have no clue what to say to you. They do not know if they should ask how you are, because they fear that bringing it up will cause you pain. On the flip side, some fear that if they do not ask how you are, you will consider them rude or callous. Given that choice, it is far easier for them to shrink away. Little do they know that the worst thing they can do is disappear on you.

But that is precisely what happened at my place of employment. When you work with more than 70 people, somebody is always asking you to go to lunch, or for a cocktail after work. After the news broke about the cancer, those invitations from the lawyers and staff came to a screeching halt.

I mostly ate lunch by myself. Being alone with your thoughts, especially when those thoughts are dark, is not good. When you are suffering, it is best to be around people, especially those who love you and won't let you get down. Let them love you. It helps you and them. A win-win for all.

What I should have done was to stick my head into their offices and simply said "You need to go to lunch with me." It would have put them at ease, and more importantly, given me a break from my dark thoughts.

Sometimes, when it seems things couldn't possibly get any worse, an angel appears. At the seven-month mark, I had a court appearance on a day when we were supposed to be at Stanford for her monthly examination. I called opposing counsel to ask if we could reschedule. It was just a motion, not a trial. This kind of request is almost always granted. But he said no. He was representing the person suing, known as the plaintiff, and maybe thought I was looking for needless delay. So I explained my circumstances. How my wife was sick with cancer, and how we had to fly out to California every 30 days to see a doctor there, because of the complication of pregnancy. Incredibly, he still said no, telling me to get another lawyer at my firm to cover the hearing. Nice, huh? Is it any wonder why most of the world hates lawyers?

A very sympathetic and wonderful female court bailiff made the continuance happen, so I could make the trip. When she told the judge what had happened, he told that lawyer that if he ever wanted to practice in his courtroom again, he would have to apologize to me and my wife, *in writing*. I got that letter, along with an apology on the phone. And I believe it was sincere, that the guy had genuinely felt regret about his behavior.

Around the same time, I made a big mistake. I waited and waited for one of the partners at the firm to tell me I could take the five or six months to be with my wife and newborn child in California with pay. It never happened. As Forrest Gump said, "Stupid is as stupid does."

I should have gone in to one of the top partners and said, "My wife is in a fight for her life. She and my newborn child are going to be 2,300 miles away from me for five or six months unless you help me by giving me a paid leave, please! I need to be with her, and I need to be paid so I can support my family."

So what could he say? No? If he did, I could go to the next partner, and the next one, until I found a sympathetic ear. But I never asked because I was afraid I would lose my job. Competition was keen among the younger lawyers, and not everyone was going to make partner. But doing nothing was the wrong move. I look back now and realize they were not going to fire me. If they did, can you imagine if I went to the press and told them what happened? Once again, fear prevailed.

Employers should look after employees who are suffering from cancer or any other serious disease. Caretakers and the non-cancer significant others are under tremendous amounts of stress. I shudder when I think back to this time frame, because I was a lawyer representing people and corporations in court, at times totally exhausted from stress and anxiety.

In the United States, we now have the Family Leave Act, which allows an employee to take time off to care for a seriously ill spouse or immediate family member, but without pay. That no pay rule eliminates most Americans from being able to take advantage of that law.

During your time of crisis when you feel dark thoughts creeping into your head, stay connected to people who love you. And know that there will be people who will show you love, people you don't even know, when you least expect them. I will never forget that bailiff. She didn't know me, but she spent 10 minutes telling me she would pray for me and that she would have people in her evangelical church pray for me, my wife and my unborn child. And she assured me that miracles happen. I hung on her every word. I was so upset with the thought that I was not going to be able to accompany my wife on this critical visit, and presto! There appeared this angel to rescue me.

LOOKING BACK/LESSONS LEARNED

➤Take comfort in knowing these angels will appear. Maybe it's the doctor, who truly cares for you by spending extra time explaining how you will get better. Maybe it's your pastor or best friend who keeps your head above water. I am convinced that there are no coincidences—people will appear and lift you up. And often as not, they will be strangers.

➤If you are the non-cancer spouse, or significant other, ask for time off from your job. Many employers will do everything they can to accommodate your needs. The Bible makes this point: "Ask and you shall receive, seek and you shall find, knock and the door shall be open unto you." You will never get what you don't ask for.

Chapter 12

That trip to Stanford in January was critical. The doctors there told us that the goal was to get our pregnancy to the seventh month, so the child would have a strong chance at life. However, if the X-ray showed cancer in my wife's chest, the baby would have to be induced, so that my wife could begin treatment immediately. We held our breath during the fifth and sixth month visits, but the news was good. The same held true at the seventh month visit—nothing on the X-rays. So the decision was made to go full term.

Finally! Good news to tell, to her parents especially and her siblings and friends. Our baby was hopefully going to have the same shot at life as any other full term baby.

We found a house to rent shortly after that trip. Two bedrooms and one bath, said the realtor. Twelve hundred square feet, at the ridiculous price of $3,000 a month plus utilities. It was the cheapest we could find near the hospital. But how we would pay for it, I had no idea.

Back home in Kentucky again, we struggled to be normal. We even took Lamaze classes, sitting on a floor with a whole bunch of happy, giddy couples. I remember their faces, seeing how the two of us had been just a few months earlier. At such moments, I almost wanted to get up and leave. On the other hand, I knew that we might not have the chance to experience the joy and excitement of pregnancy ever again.

Try as I might to fight them back, dark thoughts kept entering my mind. How cruel would it be if we kept going to these classes, only to have something wrong with this child because of the cancer, the X-rays, and the unimaginable stress that she was enduring?

Having two lives on the line was overwhelming. And when you're overwhelmed, fear and anxiety start creeping in. When you're dealing with that combination, it's hard to see the sun shining on a cloudless day.

Ever the tough guy, I kept it all in. She did, too. And our fear and anxiety kept us from talking.

In late January I went to visit the bank, to make certain that I could forgo paying our mortgage on our home in Kentucky. I explained to this vice president guy once again that the house in Palo Alto we were renting was over $3,000 a month. Sure, he said, no problem. Best wishes.

Another angel appeared on the horizon one month later. I was prepared in February to drive my car to California, so when the time came for my wife to be treated at Stanford, she would have a way to and from the hospital. A buddy of mine from New York, who had transferred to Kentucky for work and who lived nearby, called and asked how I planned to get my car out there. When I told him, he would have none of it. What happens, he asked, if you're on the road and the baby comes early? You'll miss the delivery, he said. He would not take no for an answer.

So what did he do? He took a vacation week and by himself, drove our car all the way to California, and flew back. Now that is a friend! We played softball years earlier in New York. He played second base, and I was the shortstop. Ask anyone who knows baseball—those two players have to work in concert. That bond stayed with us. God bless my friend, Tom Krpata, who was another angel who appeared in our time of need.

LOOKING BACK/LESSONS LEARNED

➤ At this time in my life, and for the first time in my life, I was consumed with "what ifs." I couldn't see through the darkness that had enveloped me. I had come to expect the worst. It wasn't like me, not at all. I had always been an optimist. I always thought things would work out. After all, I had the faith and courage to leave home and give law school a shot, knowing I did not have the money to last more than six or seven months. So what happened to that Irish optimist? Where did he go? Negativity is like Kudzu, an invasive vine that spreads at the amazing rate of 150,000 acres a year, choking out all other vegetation. Once it takes root, there's hardly any stopping it. Another reason to seek help.

➤ Thinking positively and staying positive is key. If your spouse or family member has cancer, you have to be healthy in order to help your loved one regain his or her health. If you have the cancer, your doctors have already talked to you about the importance of positive thinking.

➤ So how do you stay positive? Read your Bible. Go to a bookstore or the library and sample some authors who preach the power of positive thinking. Read one or more of Dr. Bernie Siegel's books to learn how important your thoughts are, and how love can see you through. Back then, I was very much a former New Yorker. We are first cousins to Missourians when it comes to skepticism. Although it would be years before I would discover the healing power of such writings, long after the worst of the emotional damage had been done to my marriage, they truly did help me.

➢ You are never too old to learn, and if you can embark upon this process now while you are in the midst of a crisis, you will benefit greatly by learning to stay positive and living in the present. As the Bible says in the sixth chapter of Matthew, "Do not worry about tomorrow, for tomorrow will worry about itself."

➢ At such a bad time, what keeps you from falling apart? Your family and your friends, hopefully. But above all, keep the faith!

Let love and faithfulness never leave you
Bind them around your neck
Write them on the tablet of your heart

Trust in the Lord with all your heart
And lean not on your own understanding
Proverbs 3:3-5

Chapter 13

At 6:30 a.m. on Wednesday, March 4, 1987, her water broke. She was so excited, and I was a wreck. I guess it was another example of what cancer couples go through, not being on the same page. As she calmly prepared for the 20-minute trip to Christ Hospital, I kept thinking, *what if something is wrong with this child?* On the drive, she talked about boy's names while I worried that this event would trigger the beginning of the radiation, and her move to California. I worried, too, about how she could summon the strength to fight her disease should something turn out wrong with the baby. We occupied the same car, but we were many miles apart.

How I regret letting my fear overshadow the excitement of that day. I simply could not stay in the present.

On that day, an extraordinary moment occurred. The birth in itself was extraordinary, of course. But there was something else. At one point during labor, I noticed what seemed like a dozen nurses gathered in the delivery room. What now? I saw a nurse with a clipboard and figured she was in charge. I coaxed her to the back of the room and asked if she was keeping something from me. Was something wrong? What were they anticipating? What were all these people doing in here?

She apologized. No, she said, nothing was wrong. It was just that the nurses understood the situation. They had heard about the woman with cancer who had put her baby's life ahead of her own, and they had come into the room to pray for a healthy child.

Our baby was a perfect little girl. We named her Elizabeth. There were many tears of joy in that delivery room.

That night after everyone left and my wife was sleeping, I sat alone in the hospital chapel. I felt pulled in so many directions. On one hand, I was a father for the first time. On the other, I had a very sick wife. I was afraid for her and for myself. I had no idea how we could afford the exorbitant monthly rent on the house I'd found in Palo Alto, the house where my wife and daughter would stay during the five months of my wife's treatments at Stanford.

On top of that, we had a mortgage at home in Kentucky and car payments. My income was not enough, and the firm would not give me paid leave. Who would I get to stay with my wife while I was working 2,300 miles away? How do you ask people to take a week off from work? How would I pay their airfares? All these same questions had been swimming in my mind for months, and I still had few answers. I kept them inside, thinking my wife had enough to worry about. It was still another of the ways that cancer eats away at a couple, although I didn't know it at the time. Fear shuts down communication.

We had just a few days at home with Elizabeth. Family and friends came to see our beautiful daughter. We went through the motions, but like a death row inmate who counts the hours to the day of reckoning, we wanted to stop the clock, so we could enjoy the days together as a family. It was amazing just to sit on the couch holding my child, staring at her face as she slept. But I knew that in just a few short days, I would be thousands of miles away from her, and that pain was unbearable.

Twelve days after Elizabeth was born, the three of us were on a plane to California. Sadly, we left on my wife's birthday. The owners of our rental home were waiting when we arrived. They were a wealthy couple in their 70s, totally fit, totally Californian. The realtor who had helped me find the house was there, too.

What happened is as vivid in my mind's eye as if it happened 10 minutes ago. When we walked in with our infant daughter, my landlord's wife was not happy. "Why would you take a newborn on a cross-country flight?" She had no idea of our circumstances. My wife, who had been worried sick about taking Elizabeth on such a long journey in a pressurized cabin, burst into tears. She handed Elizabeth to me and ran out the door. The realtor quickly told the couple about the cancer, the pregnancy that never should have succeeded, the misdiagnosis, the upcoming treatment at Stanford, all of it. With that, my landlord's wife also began to cry and ran out the door after my wife. Then the realtor looked at the tears forming in my eyes, became upset, and bolted out the door after both of them.

I stood there with Elizabeth in my arms looking at my new landlord. He looked at me. After a long awkward silence, he suggested I put Elizabeth in her stroller and the three of us take a walk. So off we went.

He asked how I planned to pay the rent. I told him he had nothing to worry about, that he would be my first payment each month. He asked what I made as an associate in a Cincinnati law firm. Instead of answering, I told him again that the rent would be the first bill I would pay each month. With that, he explained that he had all the money and all the homes he would ever need, and that my rent should be the last bill I pay each month. I guess he could tell I wasn't making a mountain of money.

Over the next week, he and his wife told everyone at their large Episcopal church about us, literally taking to the pulpit to tell our story. Perfect strangers began showing up at our door with covered dishes, casseroles and all kinds of homemade meals. This went on for months. Meanwhile, our landlords became regular visitors, helping with Elizabeth and looking in on us. I had never experienced anything quite like this outpouring of God's love. And there was more to come.

One day while my wife was undergoing another round of radiation treatments, I found myself sharing a waiting room with another 70-something Californian. I don't remember what precipitated it – I was lost in the fog of everything that was happening – but the man turned to me, looked me in the eye and said, "Son, looks like you're having a bad day. What's the problem?"

Without pausing to consider why he was there, I launched into a rant about my latest calamity. Compared to everything else, it was a small thing. But it was another knot in an already tangled rope. This time it was my car. It was constantly stalling, even at 30 to 40 miles an hour. I told him all about it. How a local dealership had worked on it four times and hadn't fixed it, how they were going to have someone in from Michigan to look at it, the whole sorry tale. I told him about my wife, and how we were taking taxis back and forth from our rental home to Stanford, and how she was scared to death that she might vomit in the back of a cab.

Then it was time to leave. I stuck out my hand, introduced myself and apologized for venting. I also apologized for forgetting my manners and not asking why he was in the waiting room. It turned out his wife was also being treated for cancer. It didn't look like she was going to make it, he said. He gave me a big hug and told me to keep fighting. On the way out the door, I realized I needed to change my attitude about "left coast Californians."

That evening, the doorbell at our rented home rang. I opened the door, and an Asian woman handed me a set of car keys. She gestured to a brand new Cadillac in the driveway. "Mr. Sugg wants you to have this car until yours is fixed," she said.

Without another word, she turned and walked toward a second car with a driver waiting. I hurried after her, caught her by the elbow and asked, "Who is Mr. Sugg?" She explained that he and I had met earlier that day in the waiting room while our wives were undergoing radiation. I didn't know how to thank her. I asked her if I might contact Mr. Sugg. She gave me his phone number, then climbed into the back seat of the waiting car and pulled away.

I walked back into the house and called the number. When Mr. Sugg answered, I was so emotional at first I could barely speak. I thanked him repeatedly, and we had a conversation about the things we had in common. He asked if I played golf. I said that I did, and he invited me to meet him at his club a few Saturdays later. We became good friends, and would remain so until his death fifteen years later.

It's just an example of the many out-of-the-blue solutions that presented themselves time and time again to the challenges I faced. Where I would see a problem with no resolution, God provided a way.

It was a Godsend, for instance, that my wife's employer, Delta Airlines, made it possible for me to fly for free every weekend to be with her. I would work Monday through Thursday, then leave Thursday night for San Francisco. On Saturday, I would drive the person who had stayed with my wife and daughter during the week to the airport. Then I'd pick up the new helper on Sunday, being sure to teach that person the route from the house to the hospital and back. That was key because my wife got sick almost as soon as each radiation treatment ended and was in no condition to provide directions. On Sunday night, I'd catch the red-eye back to Kentucky, land the next morning at 6:15, shower, shave and go to work. I was stretched to the limit. Still, I wasn't the one with cancer.

LOOKING BACK/LESSONS LEARNED

➢ All those weeks of classes, and guess what – I forgot the Lamaze bag! That was my only job, and I blew it. Worrying about whether the child would be healthy, followed by the joy of seeing the birth of a beautiful child (a perfect 10 on the Apgar!), followed immediately by the experience of holding her, then realizing that for the better part of five months, I would be apart from them both – I was riding an emotional whipsaw. I began to feel intense sorrow at the thought of being separated from my wife and child for extended periods. All because my bosses at the firm wouldn't give me time off from work. Then again, I hadn't asked for it. I was afraid of losing my job. How foolish I was to not even venture the request.

➢ In such a situation, maintaining your composure and better judgment can be nigh on to impossible. The situation clouds everything you do. Maybe you get tense in the waiting room as your loved one is getting a chemo treatment. You try, but you cannot even focus on a six month old issue of People magazine. You sit, you stand, you pace. Or maybe you're the one in the chemo room, sick with the thought that your whole family is in turmoil over your illness. You know it is not your fault, but you feel like you should apologize. If any of this sounds familiar, take comfort in knowing that you are not alone. What you are feeling is normal and understandable. You each feel the way you do because you love the other person. Because you care so much. Because you're worried more about the other person than you are about yourself.

➤Lean on that. Make a vow that because of that bond, that love, that relationship—you are going to take care of yourself. If you are the non-cancer spouse, exercise and relax as much as you can, so you can give your loved one the maximum support possible. If you are the cancer patient, instead of worrying about your loved ones, simply let them love you.

➤Think of all of the people in the world who have attended 12-step programs, whether it be for gambling, drug addiction, alcohol, whatever. Those organizations talk to addicts about surrendering to a higher power. Of course, they have all different types of people coming through their doors. Christians. Muslims. Jews. Hindus. Agnostics. And even atheists. Many of those organizations will tell these folks desperate in need of help that it takes your higher power to get through. Back then, I believed in God, but I had no relationship with Him beyond a superficial level. What a shame, too, considering I had attended 12 years of Parochial school, was an altar boy and a reader at Mass. My prayers were all rote, rarely heartfelt. I really had no idea how to pray. I didn't have that personal relationship. I now see that if I was in closer touch with my higher power, my God, and if I had a stronger belief system to lean upon, I would have coped far better. I believe my marriage would have survived. You may have friends and family, but so many struggles come in the dark of night. That is your talking to God time—time to be listening for His answers.

➤So when nighttime comes, and you are alone with all your dark thoughts, opening a Bible will help. Open it to wherever, and see what you find. I just opened mine as I was writing this, and it fell open to the fourth chapter of Psalms, where I found these lines:

> *Answer me when I call to you,*
> *Oh my righteous God.*
> *Give me relief from my distress;*
> *Be merciful to me and hear my prayer…*
> *I will lie down and sleep in peace,*
> *For you alone, oh Lord,*
> *Make me dwell in safety.*

Chapter 14

During the first six weeks of my daughter's life, I was home alone during the week, more than 2,000 miles away from my family. It was then that the seething inside me began. I knew my place was by my wife and daughter's side, but we had to have an income. Each morning when I went to work at the law office, my chest would tighten. I despised those men who knew my sick wife and daughter were in California, and could care less.

I would arrive on Monday exhausted after the red-eye from California, and caffeinate all day to stay awake. On Tuesday, I was still trying to shake off jet lag. I called my wife every night before I went to bed, but really couldn't get her to say much. There were these 5 or 10 seconds of silence when I would wait for her to say something. When the call ended, I would worry, wishing I could be there with her. And how I missed holding my little girl! Those days started me on a slow but steady downward slide.

The weekly routine in California was radiation in the morning, followed by the return to the house, fighting nausea for a few hours, then sleep. She tried to coordinate her nap with Elizabeth's, so there was quiet in the house. Because of the radiation, Elizabeth could not be breast-fed, which upset her mother a great deal.

I received quite an education about how nerve racking parenting could be during those first few weeks. It was time for Elizabeth's first immunization, and for medical reasons, my wife was told not to attend. So on Friday I took her to the pediatric department at Stanford, where a very kind doctor and staff were waiting. When we were called back to a treating room, my heart was beating rapidly. She was so little, so precious…

Then the doctor walked in. And with him came the tray with the needle on it. He started to ask how the cancer treatment was going, but I could not stop looking at that large needle, imagining it piercing my tiny daughter's body.

"Are you okay, Kevin?" he asked.

"Not really," I replied.

He smiled, and told the nurse to walk me back to the waiting room. She took the baby from my arms, and when I tried to stand up, well…remember Gumby? That little rubber man? I suddenly had Gumby legs.

I think back to that moment and smile. As a fireman in the 1970s, I went running into burning buildings when others were running out. Yet the thought of my baby girl being in pain caused my legs to turn to jelly. When you love somebody, you find feelings and emotions you never knew you had. That is a good thing.

At the end of April, the first of the three-part treatment— the radiation to my wife's neck and chest—was completed. She was given ten days to rest, for the toughest part of all was still to come—the laparotomy surgery. We both dreaded it for a number of reasons. The surgery was brutal in terms of the length and depth of the incision, and how painful the recovery would be. But the thing we feared the most was the news it could bring. Her cancer was initially diagnosed by Stanford as stage two. However, the doctors told us that if it had spread to her abdomen, it would be a fight for her life. Which made the instructions to "Go home and rest" seem amusing. But it was good to have my small family back home in Kentucky, even if for only that short time.

When it was time to fly back to California, we decided to leave Elizabeth with her grandparents. The plan was that my wife would finish packing while I drove Elizabeth to her grandparents' house. That goodbye between mother and child … there are no words. She was so weak from six weeks of intense radiation, commencing immediately after she had given birth. Now, facing such a serious surgery, I knew my wife wondered if she would ever see the baby again.

On the way to her parents, I had to stop and pull over. I could not see through my tears. I wanted to scream. It was so unfair, so wrong. I could not understand how a loving God could have allowed that moment to happen. In the next breath, I prayed to that very same God that she would hold that baby again and again, for years to come.

LOOKING BACK/LESSONS LEARNED

➢I started ignoring certain bills, because I had no money to pay them. I was paying airfares for others who flew to California to help while I remained home to work Monday, Tuesday, Wednesday and Thursday. I worried if she would survive. I began to worry that she and my child might not have a house to return to after the treatment was over. More worry. More anger. Why didn't I ask to borrow money? How easy it would have been to simply ask, sign a promissory note, and accept help to take the massive burden off my shoulders. Heed this, please! Remember, the most amazing man to walk this earth accepted help not once, not twice, but three separate times as he carried His cross up the hill to save us all.

➢Once again, in the midst of such a dark time, an angel appeared in a nurse's uniform. When I was escorted out of the needle room and back out to the waiting area, the nurse held my arm, smiling all the way. As said, I was a little wobbly, but puzzled by her smile. When she sat me down, this woman, twice my age, kissed me on the cheek, and whispered, "You're going to be a great dad." What a tender moment from a loving woman! To all of you in the medical profession, what a difference you make by caring! The power you have to lift people up is huge. And even a whisper of encouragement from anyone, medical professional or not, can make a vast difference for the better.

Chapter 15

Before we knew it, we were back at Stanford. We met with the surgeon prior to the procedure, along with a doctor in training, called a resident. After explaining the surgery and the risks, he made it clear he was open to any questions we might have. I asked the first one delicately. Had he ever performed this particular surgery? He smiled and said, "Yes, hundreds upon hundreds of times – probably more than five hundred times." A wave of relief washed over me. I asked several more questions, and he answered each thoughtfully and completely, taking more time than I would have expected.

After he left, the resident physician remained to ask if I knew anything about the guy that just left the room. I didn't, other than the fact that he knew how to make a good impression on a husband scared to death.

"He's our chief of surgery," the resident said. I was shocked. The number one guy! Then again, I knew everyone at Stanford was pulling for my wife. They appreciated what she had done and the risks she had taken for her baby. Still, I couldn't help but be grateful. There we were, two kids from Kentucky, going through the hardest time in our lives, but getting top treatment at the top hospital from the top docs in oncology, radiation therapy and surgery.

The surgery seemed to last a couple of decades. When it was completed, I was called into a little room, to wait for the doctor. After yet another eternity, in he came. He didn't have to say a word. I could see in his face that the news was bad. He told me the cancer had invaded her spleen. It was stage three, which meant it had spread.

It was all I could do to walk back the few steps to the waiting area. During the surgery, I sat next to a Jewish woman from New Jersey. After getting the bad news, this dear woman—a perfect stranger—let me put my head on her shoulder and cry for half an hour, stroking my head. After collecting myself, I returned to the house, and then made the calls to my wife's parents and brothers and sisters. More calls, more bad news to deliver. Her dad cried on the phone. That killed me. Everyone knew she was now in a fight for her life. All doubt of that had been removed. When I hung up from the last call, I was numb, in a tiny house alone, far from home.

After an extended stay in the hospital, my wife was sent home to Kentucky for a few weeks to rest and heal. Coming home to that beautiful miracle child sure did help her, and seemed to take her mind off the pain she was experiencing as a result of the surgery.

After a recovery period that seemed to me to be far too short, the next round of radiation began—six weeks to the stomach and pelvic region. The assaults seemed so relentless, so never ending.

Meanwhile, some ugly business was unfolding back in Kentucky. Before we moved to California, I previously told you that I visited the bank that held our mortgage to explain that I would be unable to pay the mortgage while we were renting the house in California. That nice vice president with whom I had spoken had assured me the bank was willing to let me go without a payment while we were in California.

Well, on a Tuesday night three months into the treatment, when I was alone in my home thousands of miles away from my wife and child, the doorbell rang. It was the sheriff – a man I knew. As he handed me the eviction papers, his eyes filled with tears. He muttered that he was sorry. I looked at the complaint and saw that a lawyer from the firm representing the local Catholic Diocese had signed the papers. The irony was deep and wide: a pro-life law firm was taking steps to have us booted out of our home – including my courageous wife, who in my mind deserved to be the poster girl for the pro-life movement.

Another night, the repo man came for my car. Lucky for me I was up late watching TV and heard his tow truck. I chased him off and hid the car in a neighbor's garage. That was definitely a low point. I realized so clearly that the world is full of people who could care less what someone might be going through, because money comes first. I will never become one of those people.

LOOKING BACK/LESSONS LEARNED

➤When your lenders send a sheriff to come for your house, and sue you for all the world to see; when the repo man comes to haul away your car and leave you standing at the bus stop the next morning; when you're the man of the house and cannot pay your bills, you feel like a total failure. If that sounds sexist or straight out of the Ozzie and Harriett era, my apologies. It is simply the truth.

➤As the non-cancer spouse, you want your partner to be able to concentrate on getting well and not spend one second worrying about anything else. You want to take care of everything, including the house, children, work, and the bills. You want to provide the best medical care available. But what happens when the bills outweigh your income? That is not your fault, is it? Of course not. So why did I feel so broken, so inadequate? Is it the result of thousands of years of learned behavior, handed down from one generation of men to the next? Is it in the strands of male DNA? I don't know. All I know is that I wish I had somebody to tell me it was not my fault, because *it was not my fault*. I wish I hadn't threatened that repo man with my fists – he was only doing his job. For all he knew, I was just another deadbeat who didn't pay his bills on time. Looking back, I think I understand why I felt the way I did. I can see that by dropping the thousands of years of learned prideful behavior, my problems could have been easily solved. I should have talked to somebody, like a pastor. I should have gone to any number of people to ask for money, as I have told you in previous chapters. I should have sought counseling, so that someone experienced could have told me that everything I was feeling was normal, not my fault, and not without solutions.

Chapter 16

The next round of radiation began—six weeks to my wife's stomach and pelvic area. It seemed so relentless, a never ending series of attacks from all sides, totally expected but totally unpredictable at the same time. Human beings are not well equipped to endure extended periods of stress.

Chunks of her hair fell out. She weighed less than 100 pounds, and her skin on her neck and chest was burned from the radiation. I could hardly bear to look at the scar across her midsection—it was such a stark reminder of the extreme pain she endured in having her gut opened up. But she kept fighting.

I was breaking down, but in a different way.

About three weeks before her treatment finished, I left work on a Wednesday, right around 7 p.m. My exit off the interstate was some seven miles from my office. The next thing I knew, I was looking at an exit sign that told me I was nearing Lexington, Kentucky, some 60 miles past my exit.

Who had been driving that car? I have no idea. I pulled over to the side of the road and shook uncontrollably. I wondered how I could have driven that far without realizing it. I was lost, swept up in my thoughts and fears.

I drove to the next exit, bought a soda at a gas station, and tried to collect myself. I realized I easily could have killed myself or some other driver, due to my complete inattentiveness to my driving. I could have left Elizabeth to grow up without a father.

I realized on the way home that everything that had happened was overwhelming me. Yet I thought I could make it to the finish line. Think about it—even the fact that I had missed my exit by 60 miles was not enough of a red flag to convince me I needed professional help, or just open up to someone, anyone about what was going on inside my head.

I look back and think of all the things I could have missed in Elizabeth's life – the night she became prom queen, her graduation day from college. I shake my head when I think of how that event was not enough to persuade me to see I couldn't handle this burden on my own.

Finally, the day came—the final radiation treatment. The plan was for my wife and her mother to fly home with the baby. My job was to clean and close the house, then drive the car back to Kentucky. On the way to the hospital, all these responsibilities were swirling in my brain. While waiting for her treatment to finish, a nurse asked me to meet with some people down the hall.

There I was introduced to a sociologist, a psychologist and two interns who told me that we would never have another child. In their experience, no woman ever conceived a child after receiving the type of pelvic radiation my wife endured. The message was if we wanted another baby, we should get on an adoption list. My first thought was how fortunate we were to have Elizabeth.

The conversation took a turn that was both more immediate and more serious—to the high frequency of divorce among what the four health care professionals referred to as "cancer couples." They mentioned statistics to show that divorce rates among cancer couples are far higher than with those who don't experience cancer. I nodded thoughtfully, to convey to them that I was giving their advice serious consideration. But inwardly, I thought, "Yeah, well, that might be true of other couples, but not us. We've been to hell, and we are getting out today." But as I had done during practically every other instance through our ordeal, I kept my thoughts to myself.

They cited statistics that showed cancer patients typically go through several stages of grief, but that I may have skipped over a stage or two because the spouse who doesn't have cancer is swept up in what they called "the care mode." Privately, I dismissed their concerns. I was in no mood for more bad news. My thinking was that if we could make it through the past year, we could handle anything. I just wanted to go home. I wanted my life back. I wanted my wife back. And I wanted to bring my daughter home for good.

But I humored them. I thanked them for the wonderful treatment we received, and left. I should have listened much more closely to their advice than I did.

After dropping off my mother-in-law, wife and baby at the San Francisco Airport for the final flight back to Kentucky, I began the long drive home. As the miles whirred past between California and Northern Kentucky, I thought back on those terrible months. I thought of the acts of kindness that sustained us during that time. I thought of all our friends and relatives who had taken a week off from work or had used vacation time to look after my wife and daughter. I thought about a lawyer buddy who out of the blue, sent us a $2,000 check to California with a note that read, "Thought you could use this." I was overwhelmed. I cried right there at the mailbox. At that point, I was dead broke with weeks to go before my next paycheck.

The outpouring of help from friends and strangers alike was amazing. I thought of folks in California who had given so much help, including the wonderful people at Stanford University Hospital. I thought of my chance meeting with Mr. Sugg and the generosity he showed, along with the parishioners at my landlords' church who prepared home-cooked meals for us. As the white lines on the interstate drew me nearer to home, I also thought of the law firm I was returning to, the people who had never offered me a paid leave of absence in our family's time of need. I knew I had to find a way to get out of there and find other employment.

I arrived home Sunday night exhausted. The next morning, I went to work. At 10:00 a.m., I was notified that my mid-year review would take place in an hour and a half. Everyone in the office was well aware that I had just driven across the country. What were they thinking?

Three partners attended the meeting – my mentor, a partner for whom the firm was named, and a corporate attorney who had never had a callous on his hand and wouldn't know a shovel from shinola. At the end of the review, the corporate lawyer acknowledged I'd had a difficult year but the firm would tolerate no more "*excuses.*"

"You had better bill some big hours over the next couple of months," soft hands told me.

In that moment, one of the predictions of the Stanford psychologist came true. The emotions that had built up over 10 months erupted like a ruptured appendix. I told soft hands that if he would kindly wait right there, I would run home and grab my 97-pound, bald, burned and three times sliced wife. I would put a wig and a dress on her, bring her back and have her personally apologize for contracting cancer and resulting in whatever loss of income he may have incurred.

He had no response for a moment. Then in a condescending tone that cut me to the bone, he allowed that perhaps he had chosen the wrong words. Then he just smirked.

I'm not a violent person. Not normally. I'd seen plenty of it growing up – in my home, on the subway and in the streets. I never failed to show up for a fight, but I didn't go looking for them either. But at that moment, it came pouring out of me. I didn't even try to control my emotions. I went for him. For the first time in my life, at age 34, I started a fist fight.

I dove over his desk, flailing. The two other attorneys pulled me back and dragged me down the hall. Another partner joined them, and the three of them dragged me to the elevator and across the street to calm me down. There on Fountain Square, with the senior member of the law firm sitting next to me, I cried like a baby. Ten months of frustration, fear, and loneliness came pouring out of me. I was flat broke. I was constantly sick to my stomach. I was officially a mess for all of Cincinnati to see. I don't know how to express how alone I felt. Over the past several months, it seemed as if so many people I thought were friends had just disappeared.

LOOKING BACK/LESSONS LEARNED

➤You can see that my failure to seek help morphed into destructive behavior that took only a few ill advised words to provoke. I had taken an oath to follow the law and I broke it in my own law office. All the emotions boiled over. Exhaustion. Humiliation. Loneliness. The despair that comes from being broke. The isolation of feeling nobody cared. The emptiness of knowing how sick and frail my wife was. I had nowhere to go, nowhere to hide. No place to find any peace. Or so I thought.

➤And how about that driving episode? I could have killed someone the night I drove more than 60 miles past my exit. If there is such a thing as a guardian angel, he or she had to have been driving my car, because my mind was so far away from the here and now. It is difficult to stay in the present when you are consumed with fear, anger and exhaustion.

➤My wife had also withdrawn into a world of silence. Like me, she wasn't getting any psychological or pastoral help. Without either of us knowing it, the seeds of our divorce were beginning to sprout. We both had been traumatized in dramatically different ways.

➤If you are the non-cancer spouse or relative or friend, and you truly want to be a rock to your loved one, you absolutely, positively must care for yourself. If you allow your emotions to consume your energy, you will have none to give. And the way you react to your surroundings depends on the emotions you feel at any given moment. If you are angry, nothing is right in your world. The fix? To find someone who can help restore your faith – someone who will remind you that it's pointless to worry about what you cannot control. So stay in the present, take care of what you can, and leave the rest to the doctors and to God.

➤ If you are the one diagnosed with the disease, resist the almost irresistible impulse to close up to your loved ones. You are not a burden! Why do cancer victims get their minds twisted into somehow thinking they are to blame? I could not get a word out of my wife, and it was killing me. More than anything, I wanted to understand what she was feeling, whether she was optimistic or pessimistic, feeling up or feeling down. How I could better help her? But whenever I asked, I ran into the brick wall of "I'm fine." More than anything, the people who love you want to help you. Let them. It's called grace. If you want them to worry themselves sick over you, shut them out. It is the cruelest thing you can do, and the most selfish. So if you are the one with cancer, think what you would do if cancer struck not you but your loved one—you would do anything for them. Don't be a martyr.

➤ Some of my softball and bowling buddies stopped calling. Same thing with my friends at work. I received fewer invitations to lunch or to socialize after work. One might think that if these people knew I was spending four days each week on my own in Kentucky, they might invite me to dinner once in a while. Only one did – a senior partner who had me over for dinner with his family on my birthday in April. Why? Because most people don't know what to say to cancer victims and their families, so they do the worst thing they can do. They say nothing. They turn away. What do you say to someone locked in a life-or-death struggle? What do you tell someone at a funeral home who has just lost a loved one?

➢A great friend shares the pain of a cancer victim and his or her family. Just being present during hard times, even in silence, shows great love, and gives great comfort to the person suffering. And if you feel you must say something and just do not know what to say, simply tell the truth—that you have no words, but you will pray for them, and you are there to help in any way.

➢Something else helps, too. A big ol' hug! The human touch is so powerful. Take the person's hand in yours. Sometimes you don't have to say much to help. I spent so much of those five months alone. People under severe stress and despair should never be alone. We humans are social creatures. We need each other, especially during the dark times.

Chapter 17

If the story ended here, with my wife's recovery and our return home with our baby, it would be a happy one. It would be an inspiring story of triumph over cancer. But it didn't end there. The disease itself, as defined by the malignant cells that ravaged my wife's lymphatic system, had been beaten. But as God knows and as we were to learn, cancer sends out tentacles that reach deep into the human psyche. When two people are involved, the damage goes that much deeper.

Surviving cancer physically doesn't necessarily mean you've survived cancer. Cancer puts its victims smack in the middle of a war between good and evil. It is, in my experience, the ultimate test of faith, of family, of friendship. It's a war against fear, despair and anger. The biggest battle of all is the struggle with loneliness and isolation. And when you are fighting this war wounded, your odds of caving in to these toxic emotions increase.

At some point in this battle, when you are literally crying out loud or on your knees next to a toilet bowl, or in your car on the side of the road shaking, most cancer victims find themselves wondering—how could a loving God put anyone through this hell? You wonder, too, where did our friends go?

Where did I go?

John Lennon once said life is what happens when you are busy making other plans. It's true. Circumstances arise and events occur that we can't understand at the time. If we're fortunate, we may only begin to understand them dimly over time. Or we may learn from our pain. In the case of my wife and myself, once the actual disease had been beaten, our relationship began sliding into a slow steady decline.

How did it happen? After what we had gone through and to seemingly survive? It would be easy to blame circumstances. No one can deny that we suffered intense trauma. We learned about the cancer when she was four months pregnant. I remember how it felt hearing her cry in the middle of the night about her growing baby and whether it would survive. Then there were the five long months of not knowing whether the disease was stage four and about to kill the both of them. Gordon Lightfoot penned a phrase in "The Wreck of the Edmond Fitzgerald" that described that weight: "Does anyone know where the love of God goes when the waves turn the minutes into hours?"

After we learned the cancer had spread to my wife's spleen, I worried whether she would see her baby grow up. So many forces were tearing away at me – the loneliness and despair of being apart from them; her scars and the burn marks; the permanent tattoos on her body that constantly reminded her of the illness; going broke and being sued to take the house; the repo man coming for the car. I had plenty of reasons to be angry, but my anger was only hurting me – and my marriage.

Before the cancer, I was never an angry man. Was I moody at times? Yes. But never angry. But I became angry and increasingly more so. It began when I found out we were in this huge mess to begin with because that first doctor had misread the slides and misdiagnosed the tumors as benign. I cannot underscore how significant that was for me. Looking back, I see the foolishness of that. It happened. There was nothing I could do about it. I should have gotten over it. But I didn't, not for years.

My anger grew when my employer refused to give me five months to be with my wife and baby. There were days when I had to pull over and find a gas station bathroom because I was on the verge of vomiting.

During her illness, when I was working, I felt I should be with her. When I was in California, I worried about looming deadlines and the excuses that were piling up with my clients.

I was angry about coming home to an empty house when I had a brand new baby. I would walk upstairs to our bedroom at night and pass Elizabeth's baby room, with the crib empty and toys untouched. I wanted to scream. Why us? Of all people, why her? I kept asking that over and over again. It was beyond my understanding.

So what do you do at times like these? Some turn to drink or drugs, or both. Some wallow in depression. Others seek comfort in someone else's arms. Some give in to their anger and lash out in violent acts. Me? I tried my best to swallow my anger, which all to often turns out to be a short cut to ulcers and a host of other physical problems.

Some are able to weather the storm because they have something to grab onto and hold, such as their God, their family, and friends, or a counsel or pastor. I am ashamed to say I had none of those. I was still relatively new to Kentucky. I had twelve years of parochial education, was elected to my parish council, and was a reader at mass while growing up in New York. But I was missing something really important. I never had a real relationship with God. I talked to God when I needed something, and occasionally to thank him for passing the bar exam or getting a good seat at a sporting event.

Of course, I already told you I was too stubborn and proud to put my feelings on the table to a *stranger*, or a touchy-feely roundtable group of metro males.

Before the cancer and the pregnancy, my wife and I spent a lot of our time together laughing. We were close. We held hands. We were a team. We had much in common, so many things we would talk about. Then the cancer came. As it gnawed away at my wife's body, my increasing anger and bitterness ate away at my spirit.

That was very evident when God granted us a second miracle and my wife again became pregnant. There was no way, according to the Stanford docs, that this could happen. The radiation had supposedly destroyed her ability to conceive. She didn't tell me right away, I guess because she was as incredulous as the docs. But the ultrasound showed our pretty little Kathleen. There she was — larger than life!

But once again, right or wrong, we felt robbed of the joy a "normal" couple experiences when expecting. This pregnancy stirred unhappy memories of the circumstances surrounding our first. While the doc assured us that previous radiation would not injure Kathleen in utero, we still worried. But we did so in silence. Her fears also caused her to withdraw even further inward.

Ah, but our Lizzy was excited about this new life growing inside her mommy's belly. There was no proverbial sack of potatoes draped over her back. She stayed in the present—and all she could think about was having a younger sister or brother. I wish our ears had been open to the important message our little daughter was trying to tell us.

Once again, on the way to the hospital to bring Kathleen into the world, we still had not decided on a name. Because we rarely talked about it. Talking about it only took us back to a time we wanted to bury forever in the deepest ocean. How sad.

LOOKING BACK/LESSONS LEARNED

➢Three years past cancer, and we still had not shared our feelings about what that dark year had done to us. Many years later, at a men's church retreat I attended, the facilitator made the point that insecurity leads to selfish behavior. I had been selfish not to talk to my wife about the turmoil I'd gone through. She knew I was suffering but had to guess exactly what was going on. Likewise, I knew she was in anguish, but she didn't let me help her through it. I seldom knew what she was thinking. And it hurt so much.

➢Had we gotten help, we could have enjoyed the miracle of this second pregnancy. We were told this could not happen. I often imagine God thinking "What is up with these two? I sent them not one, but two miracles, and rather than be joyous and grateful, they chose to live in fear!"

➢The lesson is simple. Why worry? Does it do us any good? How foolish it is to worry about things we cannot control. But we all do it, even though we all know that worry does nothing but make us sick.

Chapter 18

Our culture abounds with stories of people we deem to be winners –often revolving around those who beat cancer. We celebrate them with Breast Cancer Weeks, 10K runs to raise money, envelopes for the Leukemia Society, on and on it goes. Newspapers and television news love stories about this person or that who has stared down the Big C. For those who manage to do so, I'm genuinely happy for them.

But many more never recover. Or if they do beat the thing that invades their bodies, they succumb in other ways. Tens of thousands go to the dark side, into private worlds ruled by fear, depression and anxiety. That includes spouses and other family members.

It happened to me, and it happened to my wife. The trauma of it all – from the initial misdiagnosis, to realizing the cancer had more than a year to spread, to the uncertainty of whether our baby would ever be born, to the five months of brutal radiation treatments, and a wickedly painful surgery – proved to be too much for her. It was too much for me as well. It turned us both inside out, into people we didn't like.

When someone is diagnosed with a major illness, it sets off a series of conversations in that person's brain, all based around the same basic premise; that is, "How am I going to get through this?" The instinct to retreat is powerful and absolutely deadly to relationships. Fear, anger, sadness … these negative emotions conspire to become a toxic brew that eats away at even the strongest couples. The psychology of a serious illness and the needs of a healthy marriage are incompatible.

Our communication faucet slowed to just a drip. Both of us craved the things we used to do together, the laughter, the hand holding, and the planned time together. But neither one of us were capable of providing such an important part of marriage, intimacy. Plus we had a newborn to care for, which masked a lot of these problems that we desperately needed to nip in the bud.

I found ways to justify my behavior with relative ease. She shut me out from the day she was diagnosed with cancer, I would say to myself. So I have a right to avoid her. She hurt me. I tried so hard to get her well. I worked so hard to set up the right doctors at Stanford, and find the folks to help care for her and Elizabeth in California. I deserved a break. So it was okay to pick from a menu of avoidance behaviors, such as playing softball three nights a week, drinking with the boys, flirting with other women, taking on too much work, and overall seeking affirmation elsewhere. After all, if she wanted to be with me, she would act like it, right? She would *talk* to me.

I have the benefit now of 20/20 hindsight. I have a wife who came home hurting. Within ten months, she had endured three surgeries, a tense pregnancy, child birth, and eleven weeks of radiation. Her skin was burned, her stomach was hurting from being split in half, and her cancer tattoos that marked the radiation beams were a constant reminder of her ordeal. She needed a strong, caring, nurturing husband who could run the entire marathon of getting her back to normal, physically and emotionally.

I ran the race, and completed several key milestones. I had a lot to do with finding the right doctors, and I am proud of that. I took on the task of making certain someone was with her every week in California, to care for her and Elizabeth while I worked 2,300 miles away. I flew out every weekend, and tried my best to keep all the balls in the air at work, at home in Kentucky, and in California.

But the race is a long one, and does not end when the treatments conclude. How could I have expected that as soon as I pulled into the garage after my drive back to California, all would be back to normal, like it was before the diagnosis? I know she wanted that just as much as I did. But we were emotionally wounded, and because we did not seek help, those wounds became infected. She would not agree to get help, and I never thought I needed it. Look what happened.

Deepak Chopra teaches a great lesson about the difference between pleasure and happiness. Pleasure is fleeting, like a one-night stand, or a laugh at a bar with your friends. That stuff has a short shelf life. It is like a drug—you need more and more to get high.

Happiness is lasting. Happiness is helping others, like teaching a child to read. Happiness is having someone you can count on, who loves you no matter what. Love is the ultimate happiness.

You will lose your sense of happiness when cancer rings your doorbell, if you let it. It is hard to be happy when you are in the midst of intense suffering. You will be tempted to look for any oasis in the desert. When you are vulnerable, it becomes harder to resist that one extra drink, or extra pill from that Valium prescription, or that person at the office who wants to comfort you in a way that crosses the line.

Counseling will help keep you on the right track. It will assist in keeping you healthy and strong. You cannot go without prayer and staying connected with church and family. If you are the one with cancer, show your love to your spouse and friends by keeping them close, and sharing your feelings with them.

It hurts when I think of that man back then, the guy I used to be who failed to see behind the curtain to what was really happening. I handle setbacks much differently now. I went for counseling, albeit too late for my marriage. I sought help in raising my two daughters, but the brilliant therapist saw right through the veneer, and went to work on me. He helped me immensely. He taught me how to be a better man, and a better father. But he also made me see the stains on my shirt, the log in my eye, and how to go about real change. Going to this psychologist was the best thing I ever did, even though as it related to my marriage, it was a case of closing the barn door after the horse got out.

My wife and I divorced long after she was given a clean bill of health. It was a slow steady slide. Our selfish behaviors had walled us up in our respective fortresses. I became a workaholic, because work was safer for me than home. In my mind, I could not make my wife happy—or even laugh. I could not get her to see the glass half full. For her, it was always empty.

So I worked, and worked some more. I would leave home at 8:30 in the morning and come home around 7:45 at night or later if I played softball. Saturday morning in the summer was my golf day. In the winter, it was just another six-hour work day.

Sunday was football on TV, a few hours of work in my home library, and time with my kids.

I was avoiding her, or so I thought. In reality, I was avoiding my inability to take away her pain and fear. I was masking strong feelings of despair and deep-seated anger because cancer had singled us out, and because I could not get her to talk about the effect it had had on her.

I chased short-term pleasure because I could not find happiness. It was right in front of me in a wonderful but hurting wife, and two beautiful miracle children. But I was blinded by my own emotions, and as many religious teachers will tell you, temptation comes when you are the most vulnerable.

She knew we were going in the wrong direction, and all those dinners I missed led to the proverbial cold shoulder. She would sit outside after the children went to bed, talking on the phone. I would sit in the basement, watching TV.

For years, we lived our lives in quiet despair, tending to the children, and acting to the outside world as if nothing was wrong.

I look back now and realize we had come to blame each other. I had come to the opinion that our deteriorating marriage was completely her fault. She thought it was all my fault. It wasn't until I went into counseling several years later that I discovered the truth.

Counseling taught me she had every right to be upset with me. My long hours at work, or staying "late at work" when I was not at work, hurt her badly and contributed to her own struggle.

Sure, she had a hand in our breakup, but if I had been doing what I needed to be doing, would we be married today? It saddens me to say, honestly, I don't know for sure.

Was the cancer the sole cause of the demise of our marriage? Probably not. But I blame most of it on the cancer—and the way we reacted to it.

It's like this: One day in the early 90s, my wife called me at work to tell me that she'd been having a hard time for the previous few days closing the patio door. The day she called, she'd been outside and seen a huge crack in the bricks on the backside of our house. It started way up toward the second floor.

What caused it? The foundation had slipped off its base, called a footer. We had to call in specialists, who literally had to lift up the whole house, using huge hydraulic jacks, and put it back in place.

Cancer had caused our foundation to slip off its base. Once our foundation was jarred loose, the rest of our "house" became weakened. We never turned to specialists, so our marriage crumbled.

We went through the motions. We took care of Elizabeth and Kathleen. We went to soccer games, school plays, and parent-teacher meetings. To the outside world, nothing was wrong.

Slowly but surely, we stopped talking altogether. When we did talk, we would argue. At the very end of our marriage, we would write notes or letters to each other. That was the only way we could communicate. Then came the lawyers—and it was over. We drove to the courthouse together on the final day. After the judge had snuffed out our marriage, we held hands on the ride home.

When the music stops, the party is over. When communication ceases in a marriage—when you cannot express your angst to your spouse without fear of reprisal, it is the beginning of the end.

I have not used my wife's name in this story out of respect for her privacy. Our divorce is without question the greatest regret of my life. But the sad fact is, once we stopped battling the cancer itself, we began to drift from each other, because we still were consumed with the awful emotions the cancer aroused.

The first piece of advice for someone facing a grim diagnosis is usually, "You're going to fight this," or "Your life is worth fighting for." In his poem, *Do Not Go Gently Into That Good Night*, Dylan Thomas exhorted his dying father to "rage against the dying of the light."

Of course life is worth fighting for. We fought the good fight against the enemy as we understood it. And we did such a great job together during those brutal months. But when the fight against the physical disease ended, we were still filled with the emotions the cancer aroused within us. We won, then we lost.

The sociologist and psychologist at Stanford were right. Among couples that experience cancer and survive the disease, divorce is not uncommon. We returned home to Kentucky with Elizabeth expecting to resume our lives as if nothing had happened. We assumed life would pick up where it had left off. We were not anticipating the aftershock.

Still, some beautiful beginnings managed to emerge. Elizabeth Murphy's birth gave her mother a reason to keep fighting. Our second daughter, Kathleen Murphy, was born in April 1990. Never mind that we'd been told that conception was impossible because of the treatment she received. I called Dr. Hancock the night she was born. I could hear him choking up on the other end. He told me Kathleen's birth was a bigger miracle than Elizabeth.

So while a part of the story ends sadly, it also became the backdrop for many wonderful new starts. I see it in the faces of my extraordinary daughters, both of whom have their mother's beauty and strength. They know they're miracle children. I've told them so many, many times. I hope they carry that knowledge with them throughout their lives. Clearly, God has a plan for them.

Elizabeth is studying for her Masters, after being a research assistant at a major university, working with substance abuse patients. Kathleen is a nursing student, looking forward to caring for children. Both are in professions to help people find joy and happiness. God is within them, and what a gift He gave me to be their Dad. What a gift my wife gave me with her courage to refuse to abort Elizabeth.

LOOKING BACK/LESSONS LEARNED

➤ I hope you see now why you must get help early. God forgave me instantly for my mistakes, but it took many years to forgive myself for contributing to the demise of my marriage, and hurting the woman I loved so much. It does not have to happen to you if you heed the warning signs.

➤ When I saw the parole scene in the movie *The Shawshank Redemption*, the words of Morgan Freeman's character, Ellis Boyd "Red" Redding, hit me like a sack of hammers:

> "There's not a day goes by I don't feel regret … I look back on the way I was then … a stupid, young kid. I want to talk to him. I want to try to talk some sense to him. Tell him the way things are, but I can't. That kid's long gone, and this old man is all that's left. I gotta live with that."

My hope for you is that you don't have to live with the type of regret I have, even though I have at long last forgiven myself. I was married to a wonderful woman, and I lost her. I can't reach that younger Kevin Murphy, but I hope I can reach you.

Chapter 19

Through the writing of this story, I have to a great extent relived it. And that has been difficult, on several levels. It's made me see in ways I never understood. That is, just how traumatic that year was.

This story crystallizes the masculine struggle. Men have a hard time owning up to our emotional side. When things are out of our control, we don't usually do well. We find it difficult to ask for help.

And when we hurt somebody, especially someone we love, we find it very hard to face them.

Then there is shame. We don't know how to deal with that either. I felt shame when we went broke. It is important for women to know that a man who cannot provide for his family because of cancer or other crisis, and the bills that come with it, suffers badly.

I felt shame when I started, as the Bible says, living in dark corners. In times of extreme pain and heartache, it offers an illusory respite, with emphasis on the word illusory.

Men have a hard time believing that any good can come from exposing your emotions, especially to a "stranger" like a pastor or psychologist.

To all men reading this, know that you need someone to help you during a crisis. Ever see anyone go into battle alone? Even Rambo took along some stragglers to help him. A counselor can help you deal with the stress and pressure, and to diffuse conflict when it comes. It can help you stay away from temptation and compromise.

So do not wait. As said by William Marstow, "On the plains of hesitation, bleach the bones of countless millions who, on the threshold of victory, sat down to wait, and in waiting, died." So have the courage to lead. Learn now that the path to wisdom is humility. You can't handle cancer alone. Take it from me. I tried. I lost.

And women! I saw a comedian on TV awhile back who did this imitation. See if it sounds at all familiar.

> Husband: "What's wrong honey?"
> Wife: "Nothing."
> Husband: 'Come on, dear. You've been awfully quiet. What's wrong?'
> Wife: "Nothing. (Turning away, folding her arms)".
> Husband: "Please talk to me, hon. Please! What's wrong? Talk to me."
> Wife: "I'm fine!"

Well, you're not fine. And he knows it. So he worries like crazy until you tell him what's wrong.

The silent treatment is just plain horrible. Over time, his worry will turn to resentment. Before you know it, a line is crossed, and he stops caring. He looks elsewhere for someone who will let him make a difference. You made him feel worthless.

The key is to talk, and keep talking, about your feelings. To ask for outside help when cancer strikes. And to try to understand that if you do these things, this dreaded disease will bring you two closer to each other, and to God.

If you don't believe me, believe the apostle Paul. He was a man's man, and at one time had a physical malady, along with other challenges. He wrote about it:

> *So I wouldn't get a big head, I was given the gift of a handicap to keep me in constant touch with my limitation. Satan's angel did his best to get me down, but what he did in fact was push me to my knees. No danger then of walking around high and mighty! At first I didn't think of it as a gift, and I begged God to remove it. Three times I did that, and then he told me "My grace is enough, it's all you need. My strength comes into its own in your weakness."*
>
> (2 Corinthians 12:7-9)
> (The Message NAV Press)

It is truly remarkable the life lessons we can learn through suffering. As odd as it sounds, suffering does teach perseverance. And perseverance leads to character, which gives you the strength to forge on.

I recently read an essay by the writer Bob Weir, called "A Conversation with God," that might bring some additional perspective to the purpose of suffering. In it, God explains that he programmed his children "to be complex beings beset by challenges and struggles which would strengthen them and force them to work out the problems of their existence in order that they be worthy of their own complexity ... (Y)ou should be wise enough to know that pain is a part of life. You needn't dwell on it, but you must acknowledge it as a vital component of your humanity."

LOOKING BACK/LESSONS LEARNED

➢ I saw this on a church marquee. Give it some thought. "No one has ever choked to death swallowing pride."

➢ Understand when cancer strikes, the entire family suffers. You need to look after all involved.

➢ As odd as it sounds, I have benefitted greatly through suffering. Paul was right—it brought me to my knees, and His strength saw me through.

Chapter 20

For a long, long time, I could never understand how we could have beaten cancer, defy long odds with the birth of two miracle children, only to wind up getting divorced. After all we had been through together, how did we fall apart? I never wanted to delve deeply into that question. I was afraid of the answer.

When I managed to face those tough questions, I was shocked to learn that I was not alone. That we were not alone. So many cancer couples wind up divorced. You will never see it on TV, or hear about it at cancer survivor relays or luncheons. But it is an ugly reality.

According to a rather recent study, female gender was found to be a strong predictor of partner abandonment in patients with serious medical illness. This study, "Gender Disparity and the Rate of Partner Abandonment in Patients With Serious Medical Illness" was published in the November 2009 issue of the journal *Cancer*. The authors, Dr. Marc Chamberlain and Dr. Michael Glantz, were surprised by their findings. "Female gender was the strongest predictor of separation or divorce in each of the patient groups we studied," said Dr. Chamberlain, who is the Chief of the Division of Neuro-Oncology at the University of Washington, and also Professor of Neurology and Neurosurgery at the University of Washington School of Medicine.

This study confirms some other troubling realities. These authors found that marital disruption may adversely affect the quality of care, the quality of life, and the outcome of treatment for the affected partner. Compared with patients who stayed together, separated patients fared more poorly, with a greater use of anti-depressants, less participation in clinical trials, more frequent hospitalizations, and less likelihood of completing their therapy.

While these doctors limited their comments to their own Neuro-Oncology practices, they were impressed by the striking gender asymmetry in the occurrence of divorce; that is, divorce appeared to occur almost exclusively when the wife was the disease-afflicted partner.

As I have detailed, I think it goes far beyond caretaking. Going broke was a huge trigger for me. Not being able to fight this monster harming and hurting my wife was another. The miles separating us killed me inside. And yes—a wife who would not talk to me, and who would not share her feelings with me. She kept it all inside, never sharing her fears. It hurt. It still does when I think about it.

But no matter what the reason, this dirty secret about cancer brings many people to a boiling point if you dare attempt to discuss it.

To better understand this issue, I have talked to many people who went down the same road towards divorce after a cancer diagnosis. Naturally, most of the people I talked to were women. They told me that it is hard enough to endure the suffering and indignity of fighting the physical aspect of this disease. But when their husbands began to drift away, the feeling of abandonment was too much to bear. It was hard for me to listen. The pain was still so raw for them.

And if you ask the woman's family members and friends about that significant other who left, watch out! You would think these folks were describing Adolf Hitler, or more appropriately, Judas Iscariot. I heard John Edwards' name surface numerous times. Edwards continued his quest for the office of the President of the United States while his wife endured breast cancer treatments. He then fathered a child with another woman during that timeframe, leading to a divorce, which was finalized not long before his wife died.

Edwards was vilified in the press. Women were especially vitriolic when talking about his misdeeds. I remember the water cooler comments at my own work place. They were brutal.

At her time of need, Elizabeth Edwards was abandoned, said the critics. His ego was so big, his narcissism so great, that he would not put her interests ahead of his own. After all, she was fighting *for her life*. John Edwards became the pariah he did because he was a public figure, running for the top job in the land. His life was lived in a fish bowl, and his downfall was just as meteoric as his rise.

That said, even a cursory read of the literature on this topic leads to a somewhat uncomfortable conclusion: that once the political power, tabloid titillation and media vilification are stripped away, the marriage of John and Elizabeth Edwards is another casualty of cancer. It happens all too frequently. It just usually doesn't get covered on "Nightline" and "60 Minutes."

Edwards was one of many men who could not "hang in there" while their wives suffered. But why is that? Why do men do these terrible things?

After all, men are brave, right? They fight for our country in time of war. They answer the call on behalf of people they never met. Firemen run into burning buildings at great risk to save the lives of perfect strangers.

Hmm…perfect strangers. There is no emotional attachment with people we don't know. It's no secret that men have a *real* difficulty with feelings and emotions. I found that out when I blew my knee out in a football game at age seventeen. The arthroscope was not invented then, so my knee was sliced wide open in surgery. I was in the hospital seven days. Those were the days insurance companies did not force you out of the hospital in what is now described as same day surgery.

Not once did my father come to visit me. When I asked my mother why, she tried to explain that he just could not handle it. I was skeptical. After all, he fought in World War II, and was a union truck driver in New York City. This was not a man who shied away from much.

When we read about men abandoning wives with cancer or other tragic illnesses, we are truly on the outside looking in. There's an old adage about marriage, that the only two people who know what happens in a marriage are the ones wearing the rings. It's true. In a cancer couple, it's gospel. We on the outside will never know the full story.

We simply select our villains from society's menu. But one size does not fit all.

If someone steals, they are a thief. Nobody should steal, right? In fact, it is one of the ten commandments that Moses came trotting down the hill with. But in some instances, is stealing somebody else's money or goods at least understandable?

I was once a law clerk to a wonderful and brilliant federal judge. One morning he came in not his usual jovial and upbeat self. I looked on the docket and saw that he had a sentencing at one o'clock. It was the other law clerk's case, but I looked into it. I became much more interested when people started pouring into the courthouse an hour before the sentencing. What was going on?

As it turned out, the defendant pled guilty to embezzlement. He worked at a bank, and through a very elaborate and ingenious 15 month scheme, was able to skim somewhere in the neighborhood of $70,000. When finally caught, he completely cooperated with the Federal Bureau of Investigation. They marveled as to how he was able to keep a secret for so long.

Why did he do it? As it turns out, he had a very sick child who was in desperate need of a transplant. Even with the newfound stolen money, he was driving a twelve year old car, and lived in a very old, modest house. He was not stealing to support a drug or a gambling habit. He was not stealing to live an exotic lifestyle with fancy cars or vacations. Rather, he was stealing to keep his child alive. And all those people streaming into the courthouse were there to support him, including his pastor, who gave an impassioned speech to the judge, begging for leniency.

What do you do in that circumstance? He broke the law. He stole money that was not his. If everybody who was in financial trouble due to illness started stealing, what would happen to society? But on the flip side, here was a wonderful man, a wonderful husband and father, with an impeccable work record prior to his son having kidney failure. He saw no way out, so he did something terribly wrong.

Some might say that it is much easier to be sympathetic to that banker fellow than to John Edwards. However, when a man's loved one is dealing with a disease he cannot fight, most men struggle badly in those situations. Like my father failing to visit once in the entire week I was in the hospital. My mother was furious with him, but let's face it, men and women are wired differently. I didn't get it then. I do now.

The moral is this: Try not to judge, even when it's hard. People are far more prone to mistakes when they are vulnerable and hurting. No one is saying that what that banker or Edwards did was okay. It wasn't okay. But instead of criticism or scorn, what people need more than anything else is forgiveness, love and compassion.

The bottom line is—if we love and support couples in the throes of this dreaded disease, we can hopefully prevent divorce from being another complication of cancer. But if you come upon a cancer couple that lost their marriage, don't scorn. Don't take sides. Some people unfortunately might be better off divorced.

And if you are in the middle of this cancer ordeal, be easy on your significant other, and on yourself. Remember my story and try to understand each other, and the feelings involved. You both need each other. You can both comfort each other. Share your feelings, and remember...by leaning on each other, you can and will hold each other up.

Conclusion

To all who helped us – all those anonymous people in California who fed us and prayed for us, to the doctors and nurses at Stanford who willed us through with their love and dedication, to the late Mr. Sugg, and my lawyer buddy who sent the check when I didn't have money to get my car out of the airport parking lot – may God's blessings flow to you all.

We're still standing. We took the blows, and we have the scars to prove it. But we're on the right side of the grass. We're still able to do for ourselves and for others.

My former wife's cancer left a big hollow space inside me. Our divorce made that hollow space something cavernous. But I have managed to fill that hollowness with a greater capacity for life, a deeper appreciation for every gift I've been given and a resolve to use what I've learned to help others get through their own hard times. That's what I gained from my suffering.

Hard times will come, you can be sure of it. The Declaration of Independence asserts our right to the pursuit of happiness, but not the guarantee of it. And nowhere in the Bible are we assured of happiness, only that we will be tested. Hard times make us what we are. The question each of us must answer for ourselves is whether we'll handle them or if they will handle us. We all need to ask for help regardless of the nature of the crisis we face. But know that the crisis will pass – and not just pass, but leave you stronger, deeper and better equipped to help others through their trials. And that, I've come to realize, is where we can find joy and fulfillment.

"You may not be interested in war," Leon Trotsky once said, "but war is interested in you." That is usually how it goes. We don't often get to pick our fights. They're usually thrust upon us. Which means we can't prepare for them. We can only react. Neither my wife nor I ever expected her to be stricken with cancer. We took the same wedding vows most couples take. We promised to stay together in sickness and in health. But what do those words really mean? Who is there to walk you through the wrenching moments, those times when you think you're done and can take no more?

You'll find no end to sources of information for dealing with cancer in the physical sense. Very little help exists to help cancer victims through the emotional toll that invariably accompanies the disease, both for the patient and the patient's loved ones.

Anyone who has ever seen someone he or she loves beaten down with disease can relate to our story. There is no emotion more natural, more visceral or powerful than the human instinct to protect those we love. Think about that, and you begin to get a sense of the toll it takes on a relationship when you can't protect someone important to you.

When I began writing this story, I asked myself what result should come of it – above and beyond the feelings of catharsis and liberation I hoped would occur from expressing the thoughts and memories that have haunted me for more than two decades in black-and-white digital files on my computer.

I came to realize that everything my family went through, every hard lesson I learned, could help others following in my experience. As personal and individual as suffering must always be, I came to see in the writing of our story a way to use the experience to smooth the way for others, so that their marriages might be saved and families and friendships kept intact.

My prayer is that you will take our story and learn to fight *against* this disease, while at the same time fighting *for* your relationship. The help you need is close by, for "He comes alongside us when we go through hard times, and before you know it, He brings us alongside someone else who is going through hard times so that we can be there for that person just as God was there for us."

I pray that you will grab hold of that loved one of yours and never let go, and that you will have the wisdom to step outside yourself and not let the darker emotions consume you. Finally, I hope you will realize we are here for just a blink of an eye and that we must use every resource available to us to emerge victorious. If you do, cancer can never defeat love. Never!

Surviving and thriving.

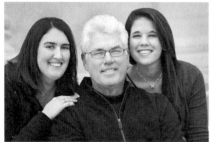

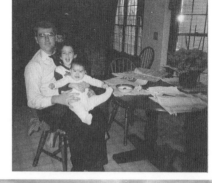

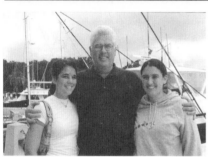

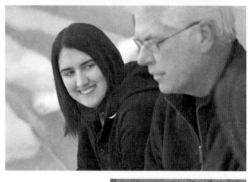

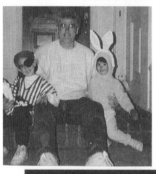

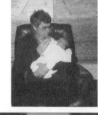

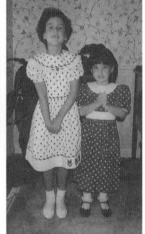

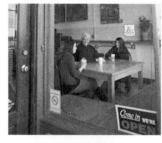

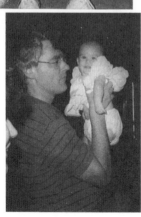

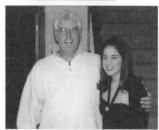

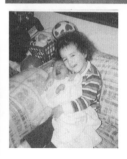

ACKNOWLEDGMENTS

This book took nearly two years to write, and never would have been completed without the love and encouragement that the following people provided to me.

To my daughters Elizabeth and Kathleen, who know my flaws and love me anyway. I am so proud to be your dad, and so proud of the wonderful young adults you have become.

To my former spouse, for her courage in putting her life on the line for her child.

To Christine Duggins, my wonderful assistant and friend, who believed in this project every bit as much as I did, and who was a tireless and enthusiastic proof reader. It would have never happened without you, Christine.

To Susan Firey, a writer extraordinaire, who kept telling me over and over that this book would make a difference. Susan, thank you for your help, and for your continued triumphs over serious health issues.

To Rick Robinson, who worked down the hallway from me…by your actions, you taught me to chase my dreams.

To my cousin Kathleen Colón, whose artistic brilliance and limitless enthusiasm helped me greatly.

To David Wecker, for your encouragement and ideas, and for helping me believe this story had to be told.

To Dick Vitale and Dr. Jame Abraham, who supported this book a year before it was published, and who do so much for those stricken with cancer.

To Dr. Bernie Siegal, cancer surgeon, author and inspiration to millions, thanks so much for writing the foreword, for your heartfelt support of this book, and for your encouragement. It is an honor and a privilege to know you.

To my wonderful publisher, Headline Books, and to Cathy Teets in particular, thank you for believing in me and this mission.

To all the people currently stricken with cancer that I have met on this journey, along with all the cancer survivors and family members I met…thank you for your inspiration, your courage, and your honesty. May God bless you all.

And most of all, to God above, from whom all good things come. Let me be an instrument of your peace.